Progress in Rational Behaviour Th

This book is dedicated to Albert Ellis

Progress in Rational Emotive Behaviour Therapy

Windy Dryden
Professor of Counselling, Goldsmiths' College, University of London

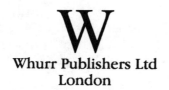

Whurr Publishers Ltd
London

© 1994 Whurr Publishers Ltd
First published 1994 by
Whurr Publishers Ltd
19b Compton Terrace, London N1 2UN, England

All rights reserved. No part of this publication may be reproduced, stored in a retrieval system, or transmitted in any form or by any means, electronic, mechanical, photocopying, recording or otherwise, without the prior permission of Whurr Publishers Limited.

This publication is sold subject to the conditions that it shall not, by way of trade or otherwise, be lent, resold, hired out, or otherwise circulated without the publisher's prior consent in any form of binding or cover other than that in which it is published and without a similar condition including this condition being imposed upon any subsequent purchaser.

British Library Cataloguing in Publication Data
A catalogue record for this book is available from the
British Library.

ISBN 1-897635-06-0

Photoset by Stephen Cary
Printed and bound in the UK by Athenaeum Press Ltd,
Newcastle upon Tyne

Foreword

Although scores of books have now been written on rational emotive behaviour therapy for professionals and for the public, few have concentrated on practical methods of how counsellors or therapists can specifically apply it to their clients. Two good books in this respect are Dryden and DiGiuseppe's *A Primer in Rational–Emotive Therapy* and Walen, DiGiuseppe and Dryden's *A Practitioner's Guide to Rational–Emotive Therapy*, which I would advise all REBT practitioners to read. As good as these manuals are, however, they omit quite a few valuable pointers which are included in the present book.

Drawing from the REBT literature, and especially from his own experience of 15 years spent using it with his own clients, Windy Dryden in the present book clearly and succinctly outlines many directives about REBT practice which virtually all therapists, including some not so rational ones, can put to excellent use. In reading Windy's 80 directives, some REBT practioners may see them as obvious correlates of its usual methodology. Fine. But most readers will find many hardheaded, realistic suggestions which they often gloss over or ignore and which this book may forcefully invite into their heads and their guts. Few readers will fail to benefit from Windy's practical teachings.

This is the first book published which uses the new name for rational emotive behaviour therapy, REBT. I think it will turn out to be not only the newest but one of the very best books about this school of counselling and psychotherapy.

Albert Ellis, PhD, President
Institute for Rational–Emotive Therapy
New York, USA

Preface

In this book I present 80 tips to help rational emotive behaviour therapists improve their practice. These tips have been derived not only from my own practice, but also from my experience as a trainer and supervisor of novice rational emotive behaviour therapists.

During the 15 years that I have been associated with rational emotive behaviour therapy (REBT), I have become increasingly involved with two major aspects of its development. First, I have been concerned to encourage people to use this system in a creative way – one which fully engages the client in an emotional experience. Second, I have been keen to base the effective practice of REBT on sound general therapeutic principles, drawing particularly on recent work that has been done on the therapeutic alliance. This latter theme crops up throughout the book, but especially in its opening section, and my thinking here has been much influenced by the work of Ed Bordin who died, sadly, in late 1992.

I have divided the tips that I discuss into a number of sections to ensure that the book is well structured. As previously mentioned there are 80 tips presented. It is no coincidence that this book is published when the founder of REBT, Albert Ellis, has just celebrated his eightieth birthday. Thus, the more sentimental might wish to see each tip marking a year that Albert Ellis has been on this mortal coil! However, REBT therapists are, in general, not a sentimental breed; so I will close this introduction by simply saying that I have dedicated this book to the one and only Albert Ellis.

Windy Dryden
London
July 1993

Contents

Foreword		v
Preface		vi
Part I	**Therapeutic alliance issues**	**1**
1	Use the concept of the therapeutic alliance	3
2	Vary your bond with different clients	4
3	Vary your influence base	6
4	Vary the extent of your directiveness over the course of therapy	8
5	Work to facilitate your clients' learning	9
6	Use the 'challenging, but not overwhelming' principle	11
7	Establish the reflection process	12
8	Use a common language with your clients	12
9	Maintain a goal-directed stance in therapy	14
10	Elicit your clients' commitment to effect change	15
11	Strive for philosophical change, but be prepared to compromise	16
12	Engage clients in the most productive therapeutic arena	17
Part II	**Educational issues**	**19**
13	Suggest that clients record and review their counselling sessions	21
14	Educate clients in the model and process of REBT and help them understand your respective roles within that process	22
15	Explain what you are doing and why you are doing it	24
16	Pay attention to clients' non-verbal and paraverbal behaviour	24

17	Teach and re-teach your clients the principle of emotional responsibility	25
18	Teach the full distinction between rational beliefs and irrational beliefs	27
19	Teach your clients to distinguish between healthy and unhealthy negative emotions	28
20	Teach your clients the importance of dealing with emotional disturbance before they learn new skills or change their environment	29
21	Teach your clients the effect of irrational beliefs on their interpretations of activating events	30
22	Teach your clients the difference between acceptance and resignation	32
23	Teach relapse prevention	33
24	Teach your clients the principles of REBT self-therapy	35

Part III Technical issues — 37

25	Be organised and structured in therapy sessions	39
26	Obtain sufficient information to help you carry out your therapeutic tasks	40
27	Keep on track	42
28	Choose the most suitable problem	44
29	Ask for specific examples of clients' problems	46
30	Work a problem through	47
31	Take care in your use of questions	48
32	Take great care in assessing A	50
33	Focus on core irrational beliefs	52
34	Look for hidden irrational beliefs in elements of your clients' verbalisations and behaviours	54
35	Allow for time-limited irrationalities in your clients	55
36	Guard against insensitivity when challenging your clients' irrational beliefs	57
37	Assess the basis for client change	58
38	Reinforce change without reinforcing your clients' need for approval	59
39	Do not be afraid to be repetitive	60
40	When in doubt, return to first principles	60
41	Be flexible in terminating therapy	61

Part IV Encouraging clients to work at change — 63

42	Let your clients' brains take the strain	65
43	Help your clients to engage in relevant change-producing tasks	66

44	Use a variety of self-help forms	67
45	Systematically train your clients to use REBT self-help forms	72
46	Negotiate suitable homework assignments with your clients	73
47	Encourage your clients to do daily self-help assignments	76
48	Regularly check homework assignments at the beginning of the next session	77
49	Build in generalisation	80

Part V Disputing   83

50	Assume that A is temporarily true	85
51	Dispute one irrational belief at a time	86
52	Keep your clients' goals in mind while disputing	87
53	Be comprehensive in disputing	88
54	Be meaningful, vigorous and persistent in disputing	91
55	Use time tripping imagery as part of your disputing strategy	93
56	Discover and use disputing techniques that work for you	94
57	Help your clients to not only weaken their irrational beliefs but also construct and strengthen rational alternatives	96
58	Encourage your clients to use a coping model of disputing rather than a mastery model	97
59	Encourage your clients to identify and dispute for themselves the irrational beliefs of others	99
60	Avoid premature and delayed disputing	100
61	Carefully distinguish between disputing questions and assessment questions	101
62	Encourage your clients to use the principles of overlearning while disputing their irrational beliefs	102

Part VI Dealing with obstacles to client change   105

63	Assess and deal with obstacles to client changes	107
64	Recognise that your clients bring their irrational beliefs to REBT	109
65	Elicit and deal with your clients' doubts about REBT	110
66	Assess and deal with your clients' misinterpretations of your disputing strategies	111
67	Ensure that your clients do not subtly undermine or counteract their new rational beliefs	112

Part VII Creativity   **113**

68	Make judicious use of referrals	115
69	Be flexible in your use of therapy sessions	116
70	Use techniques from other therapeutic approaches, but in a manner consistent with REBT theory	117
71	Vary the medium, but not the message	118
72	Be vivid in your interventions, but avoid being too vivid	120
73	Create new REBT techniques	121
74	Capitalise on your clients' pre-therapy experiences of personal change	122

Part VIII Develop yourself both personally and professionally 125

75	Identify and dispute your own irrational beliefs about your clients and the process of therapy	127
76	Beware the neurotic agreement	128
77	Seek regular supervision	129
78	Transcribe therapy sessions periodically and evaluate each of your interventions	130
79	Use REBT in your own life	131
80	Develop your own style in therapy and in life	132

References	135
Index	137

Part I

Therapeutic Alliance Issues

1 Use the concept of the therapeutic alliance

In the late 1970s, Ed Bordin (1979) wrote what I consider to be a seminal article in the field of psychotherapy where he introduced a tripartite model of the therapeutic alliance. His argument was that there are three major components of the alliance. First, psychotherapy is goal directed. Second, it takes place within a context of a developing bond or interpersonal relationship. Third, both client and therapist have tasks to do. Effective rational emotive behaviour therapy (REBT) occurs when both you and your client: (1) know what your respective tasks are; (2) can implement these tasks in the service of your client's goals; and (3) can work together in an adult-to-adult partnership. In this relationship you are both equal in humanity but you, as therapist, have greater expertise than your client in facilitating psychological change.

As you will know if you have practised REBT, work with clients often falls short of this ideal. When this happens, I have found it very helpful to use the therapeutic alliance concept to determine what has gone wrong in my alliance with my client and what needs to be done to repair the rupture (Safran, 1993).

Common ruptures in the *goal* domain of the therapeutic alliance occur when you and your client are working towards different goals, when you do not give your client an opportunity to state her goals, or when she has a hidden agenda where she surreptitiously seeks a goal which is at variance with her explicitly stated goals.

Ruptures in the *task* domain of the alliance frequently occur when your clients: (1) do not understand what their tasks are in REBT; (2) receive inadequate training from you in these tasks; (3) do not understand the relationship between carrying out these tasks and reaching their therapeutic goals; or (4) are being asked by you to practise tasks which have insufficient potency to enable them to achieve their goals. Ruptures in the task domain of the alliance can also occur because you, as therapist, practise REBT unskilfully. Such errors include: failing to prepare clients for the active–directive nature of the therapy, disputing irrational beliefs before clients understand the relationship between these beliefs and their disturbed feelings and behaviours, and unilaterally assigning homework assignments to clients, rather than negotiating them *with* clients.

Ruptures in the *bond* domain of the alliance are often, in my opinion, given insufficient attention by REBT therapists. While many clients do appreciate the typical down to earth, active–directive style of many REBT therapists, quite a few clients react adversely to this style. If this is your usual style, be aware that some of your clients will regard it as evidence of lack of caring and understanding on your part, whereas others, who may be highly reactant, will consider that you are imposing a mode of thinking on them and are taking away their much valued autonomy.

While I have dwelt at length on the importance of using the therapeutic alliance framework to understand when REBT does not go as smoothly as one hopes (or as one reads in many REBT texts!), I want to stress that it can also be used as a helpful framework to enhance the effective practice of REBT. For example, it can serve as a reminder for you to monitor the degree of congruence that exists between your own and your client's goals. It can encourage you to check whether your client understands both her own tasks and those of her therapist. It can help you to check that your client understands the relationship which exists between task completion and goal attainment. Finally, it can forcefully remind all REBT therapists of the interpersonal nature of their work and that effective REBT is not just a matter of, for example, disputing irrational beliefs or encouraging clients to use self-change techniques. Rather, REBT is fundamentally an important interpersonal relationship – perhaps more important in the minds of clients than in the minds of REBT therapists!

> **Key point**
>
> *Use the concept of the therapeutic alliance to maximise the practice of REBT and to identify and repair ruptures to the therapeutic process.*

2 Vary your bond with different clients

Albert Ellis has portrayed REBT therapists as authoritative (not authoritarian) psychological educators who actively and directively teach clients the ABC's of REBT and what they need to do to overcome their psychological problems. However, commonsense tells us that not all clients respond well to this style. Thus, it is important for you to be prepared to vary your interpersonal style of relating to clients in an authentic way if you are to maximise your therapeutic effectiveness. Key dimensions of the therapeutic bond that are relevant to REBT are: formal–informal, self-disclosing–non-self-disclosing, and humorous–non-humorous.

Let me consider the formal–informal dimension first. Whereas some clients will respond much better to you when you adopt a formal, businesslike expert style, other clients will respond more favourably to you when you adopt an informal, friendly style of interaction. To have a fixed interpersonal style with all clients guarantees that you will fail with some of them.

How do you judge which style to use with which client? My own practice is to discuss quite openly with clients what they expect from a therapist. Do they see their ideal therapist as someone who is authoritative and can teach them the emotional facts of life in a formal and businesslike way? Is their ideal therapist someone who is less formal, downplays the trappings of professionalism, and comes across more as a human being? Of course, it is important to guard against reinforcing a client's dire need for approval. However, I believe that it is usually possible for you to meet your clients' preferences on this issue without compromising your work as an REBT therapist. No matter what hunches you may have about your clients, you can only determine the *actual* way your clients respond to your interpersonal style by trial and error.

If REBT therapists are first and foremost good teachers, then they need to recognise that teaching can be done in a variety of styles. So consider whether your client will respond more profitably to a formal or an informal style and modify your own interactive style accordingly.

Some clients are deeply affected by therapist self-disclosure. I have found that sharing my own difficulties with anxiety about speaking in public because of my stammer has been a profoundly important experience for some clients. First, they learn that I have used REBT with myself to overcome my problems; second, they learn that rather than being an all-knowing fountain of rationality, I have my own difficulties too. This latter point can lead to profound learning for some clients who need to experience rather than know intellectually that their therapist is equal to them in humanity. However, to other clients, such self-disclosures either fall on deaf ears or are in fact quite anti-therapeutic. Such clients shrug their shoulders at such disclosures or indicate that they are just not interested in knowing about the private life of their therapist. These are clients who only wish to be helped by you as a non-self-disclosing therapist who emphasises expertise, not human vulnerability.

The third dimension of interpersonal style I wish to discuss is therapist humour. In REBT there are a number of concepts that you need to teach clients. With some clients you will be able to teach these concepts best if you use humour. In my experience, clients who respond well to therapist humour are, in fact, humorous individuals themselves. However, you need to appreciate that when some clients respond well to your humour, they may become overly giggly. Because they are having so much fun from therapy, they may stop taking you seriously as a viable helper. For such clients your humour turns therapy into entertainment rather than a serious endeavour.

Other clients regard therapy as very serious and consequently consider therapist humour as inappropriate, in that they may view you as a flippant person who is not taking them and their problems seriously. They may also consider you immature.

It goes without saying that when you use humour in REBT, direct it at your client's irrational beliefs rather than at the client herself. Do not assume that because you are directing your humorous remarks at your client's beliefs that she will not experience them as a personal attack. You may need to explain what you are doing before you do it.

I have argued that you should try to ascertain the interactive style to which your client responds best quite early in therapy, perhaps even in the first session. However, it is also important to elicit your client's feedback concerning how she reacts to your therapeutic style throughout therapy. Here I believe REBT therapists can learn a lot from cognitive therapists, who routinely seek feedback from clients at the end of every session about various matters to do with the session itself and the therapist's contribution to it. Asking for frank feedback from clients concerning your therapeutic style will be quite useful in helping you to calibrate your style in the best interests of your clients.

> **Key point**
>
> *Vary your bond with different clients, but do so authentically.*

3 Vary your influence base

Related to the issue of therapeutic style is that concerning which base REBT therapists should use to influence clients. REBT is unashamedly an approach to psychotherapy which seeks to influence clients to change their ways of thinking about themselves, other people and the world. As such, you need to consider that you may be successful in influencing a client from one base and unsuccessful in influencing the same client from another base.

Some clients seek out therapists with national and international reputations. Such people may seek out Albert Ellis purely because he is Albert Ellis. It could be true that if Albert Ellis taught them something anti-rational, then they might well be influenced by him because of his reputation. However, REBT therapists avoid basing their communications on an authoritarian position. We prefer to encourage clients to think for themselves and hopefully would never insist that clients think in a certain way purely because we say so. As Albert Ellis emphasises, there is a world of difference between being authoritarian and being authoritative. Thus, with clients who are impressed by your reputation as an authority, you will best be able to influence them by emphasising the trappings of expertise. This quality encourages such clients to pay attention and listen to you. They will be impressed by your writings, your qualifications and other professional accoutrements which demonstrate that you know what you are doing.

Other clients respond much better to a therapist's likeability. Such clients are not interested in what you know or your reputation but in what you are like as a person. Whereas for the clients discussed above the salient question is, 'What does this therapist know?', the questions for this group of clients are 'What is the therapist like?', 'Is the therapist going to like me?', 'Are we going to get on?'.

Be prepared to vary your influence base from authoritative expert to likeable person as far as you can without becoming unauthentic. If you are unable to modify your influence base, it is ethical practice to refer a client to a therapist who is, for example, more able to emphasise expertise.

Let me now consider three styles of teaching that are relevant to the practice of REBT: (1) authoritative, (2) laissez-faire, and (3) hypothesising.

Authoritative REBT therapists demonstrate clearly that they know what they are doing and this is, of course, related to the expert influence base previously discussed. Such therapists need to guard against being seduced into doing a lot of work for the client.

In laissez-faire teaching, the message the therapist communicates to the client is 'You do all the work and I will encourage you the best I can'. The danger for laissez-faire REBT therapists is that by being allowed to ramble, their clients will not discover rational principles by their own efforts. A laissez-faire style, however, is helpful for those clients who are highly reactant and who would react negatively to the active–directive stance of the authoritative therapist.

The third style is one that I call hypothesising. This style is similar to that advocated by cognitive therapists in their principle of collaborative empiricism. Here the message is 'Let's work together to discover the answer to your problem'. The problem with this style is that it can be somewhat hypocritical. REBT therapists work on the principle that they know, *a priori*, the kinds of irrational beliefs with which clients disturb themselves. To communicate that one can discover these afresh in a hypothesising style may well come across eventually as dishonest in REBT.

> **Key point**
>
> *Vary your influence base and avoid using the wrong base with your clients.*

4 Vary the extent of your directiveness over the course of therapy

Albert Ellis has always argued that REBT is fundamentally an active–directive approach to psychotherapy. In my experience it is difficult to practise REBT in the early phase of therapy without adopting an active–directive stance. At the start of therapy, you will need to direct your client to his disturbed feelings and self-defeating behaviours and direct him to understanding the ideological roots of his psychological problems. However, if you continue to be directive throughout therapy, you may well deprive clients of the opportunity to become more active and self-directing for themselves. Thus, consider fading the extent of your directiveness in a number of different circumstances. The first of these circumstances is when your client is making progress on a particular problem. Instead of continually directing the client to the ABCDE's of REBT, you can ask questions such as:

> 'What are you thinking not to be anxious?'
> 'How did you dispute that belief?'
> 'How could you dispute it more effectively?'
> 'How could you put that into practice?'

By asking such questions you will encourage your clients to internalise the model of REBT problem-solving in a way that allows them to utilise their own resources.

However, when your client introduces a new problem then you may resume your active–directive stance in helping him with that problem, especially if it has different ideological roots to the previous problem. My own practice is initially to teach all clients the ABCs of REBT and help them understand the role that musts, awfulising, low frustration tolerance and self and other downing play in their disturbance. When a client introduces another problem, I encourage him to direct himself to the four irrational beliefs to see which may be relevant to his newly introduced problem.

Many therapists I have supervised over the years assume that practising REBT in session 1 is the same as practising REBT in the middle or end phase of therapy. As a result, they tend not to change their level of activity and direction. This is a profound error.

Key point

Reduce the level of your activity and direction as therapy proceeds to facilitate your clients doing the work for themselves.

5 Work to facilitate your clients' learning

As I have already discussed, REBT is an educational approach to psychotherapy. Viewing REBT in this way helps you to acknowledge that your client is basically in a learning role. Therefore applying sound principles to facilitate learning is a key issue in the practice of REBT. What are some of these principles?

Pacing

The first principle is the need for suitable pacing. While some of your clients may learn very quickly, others may need you to go much slower. Therapists who are able to vary their pace to meet the learning needs of their clients, in my experience, practise REBT more effectively than therapists who have one set pace of working which they apply to all their clients.

Checking clients' understanding

Effective REBT therapists not only *teach* rational principles effectively, but also ensure that their clients *learn* rational principles thoroughly. Good teachers tell us that there is often a poor correlation between what one teaches and what students learn. Thus, particularly when you are employing a didactic style of REBT, check out what your client is learning from your didactic teachings. This does not mean, however, that when you are working more socratically you can forego this point even though the socratic dialogue involves you giving feedback to the client when she provides the wrong answer to your questions.

When I ask clients what they are learning from my attempts to teach them the principles of REBT, it often amazes me what they say. A common misunderstanding, for example, is that giving up one's musts and sticking with one's preferences means that you as a therapist are advocating a philosophy of indifference.

Encourage clients to take responsibility for their learning

At the beginning, I ask all my clients what they think my responsibilities are in therapy and what they think their responsibilities are. A number of my clients are quite surprised to be asked questions concerning their responsibility in therapy, as if they believe that their only responsibility is to turn up and listen to me as their therapist. Earlier in this book I mentioned that you can encourage or discourage your clients from taking responsibility for their own learning by the style you take as a therapist. Remember that one of your major roles as an REBT therapist is to help clients become their own counsellors. Helping them to take responsibility for their learning is an important step in their progress.

Cover material in manageable chunks

I have known REBT therapists cover too much material in a given session, with the result that the client learns less than she would have done if less material was covered. Therapists who have fixed ideas about how much material should be covered in REBT sessions tend to rush their clients and consequently interfere with their clients' rate of learning. Thus, it is important to cover only as much material as your client can usefully process and learn from.

Vary your use of bibliotherapy

It is important to use a wide range of bibliotherapy material. Clients respond in different ways to different types of self-help material and indeed some clients learn most about REBT by reading the professional literature even though they are not professionals themselves. They do so because they find self-help material either too simple or too patronising. For other clients, however, it is the case that the simpler the better: Howard Young's (1974) *Rational Counseling Primer* is at just the right level. When you are not sure which type of material to give to a client, offer her a range of books and ask her to report back which material she finds easiest to understand. Then encourage her to stick with this until she is ready to move on to something more complex.

> **Key point**
>
> *As a practitioner of REBT, you are educating your clients in healthy rational principles. As such, help them to learn these principles as effectively as you can.*

6 Use the 'challenging, but not overwhelming' principle

A number of years ago I introduced into the REBT literature the 'Challenging, but not overwhelming' principle (Dryden, 1985). While REBT therapists prefer to encourage their clients to take large steps forward and to take big risks to help them overcome their problems, such tasks which we as therapists might consider 'challenging' may be experienced by clients as 'overwhelming'. The fact that their experience may well be based on irrational thinking is not the point here. What is relevant is that if clients evaluate therapeutic tasks as 'overwhelming', they will not undertake them. Rather than trying to push your clients to do homework tasks from which they would theoretically benefit, but which experientially they consider to be too much for them, it is better to encourage them to choose tasks which are challenging. This would still encourage them to see that they are making progress, without threatening the therapeutic alliance, as would happen if you pushed them to do the 'overwhelming' task. My practice is to introduce clients to the 'challenging, but not overwhelming' principle and encourage them to choose a task which is challenging for them, given their present psychological state, avoiding, on the one hand 'overwhelming' tasks and, on the other, tasks that are 'too easy' for them.

If you steadfastly encourage your client to do tasks that she considers to be 'overwhelming' for her, you may be perceived as being overly demanding and insensitive to the client's feelings with the result that your client may well drop out of therapy. On the other hand, when you provide insufficient challenge for your client, therapy may well lose its potency.

Therapeutic change comes neither from overly pressurising a client to do something which she considers to be 'too difficult' for her, nor from being insufficiently challenging in one's approach to negotiating tasks. Rather, it occurs when the client undertakes healthy challenges to her irrational thinking.

> **Key point**
>
> *Encourage your clients to undertake therapeutic tasks which are challenging for them. Do not pressure them into attempting tasks which are 'overwhelming' for them, and discourage them from doing tasks which are insufficiently challenging.*

7 Establish the reflection process

The reflection process is set in motion when you and your client stand back from the work of REBT to reflect on it. This may be done at any point during a therapy session or more formally at the end of session as advocated by Beck et al. (1979). Additionally, it may well be helpful periodically to structure formal reflection sessions known as review sessions, to enable you and your client to review therapeutic progress and to reformulate the work that needs to be done in the future.

If you have worked with clients with severe personality disturbances, particularly borderline individuals, you will know how difficult it is to encourage them to reflect on the work that you have been doing with them, especially so if they are experiencing quite a lot of emotional upset. David Burns has noted in his recent workshops that the ability to empathise with the distress of such a client is one important bridge to helping him to reflect on any ruptures to the therapeutic alliance that may have occurred between you and which may have served as an activating event in the client's emotional episode.

My own practice is to introduce the concept of the reflection process to clients at the outset of therapy and mention that either of us may, at any time, refer an issue to the reflection process.

However you encourage your clients to reflect on the process of REBT, the important point is that talking about therapy can serve as a very useful learning experience for both of you. Clients can learn that they can influence the course of therapy and you can be helped to calibrate your interventions and interpersonal style to facilitate client change.

> **Key point**
>
> *Establish the reflection process and refer issues to it at suitable points throughout REBT. Encourage your clients to do the same.*

8 Use a common language with your clients

A number of years ago I wrote a paper called 'Language and meaning in rational emotive therapy' (included in Dryden, 1987). My intention in writing the paper was to encourage REBT therapists to consider the language they use with clients and to work with clients towards a common understanding of the concepts that they introduce. It is important to appreciate that your clients may make different interpretations of particular rational concepts than the meaning implied in such concepts. For example, take the word 'rational'. In REBT, rational means flexible, self-enhancing, empirical and logical. To clients, however, the term may mean unemotional, robotlike, a state to be avoided rather than to be desired. If you have established an effective process of reflection with your client (see p. 12), then you can discuss the different meanings of the word 'rational'. The language you use with your clients serves as an activating event which they will interpret and evaluate. Therefore, it is very important to check out with clients their interpretations of the words you use. Misunderstandings at both inferential and evaluative levels may serve as real roadblocks to therapeutic progress.

In this context, it is particularly important to consider words which point to the emotions. REBT theory keenly distinguishes between what Albert Ellis calls appropriate and inappropriate negative emotions (I prefer to call these healthy and unhealthy negative emotions). If you use feeling words in the way that they are employed in REBT theory without further explanation, your client may well become confused. Thus, it is important to explain your distinctions. For example, it is important to distinguish between anxiety (an emotion considered to be unhealthy in REBT theory) and concern (one that is considered to be healthy). However, if your clients find such terminology unhelpful, elicit from them distinctions which are more meaningful to them but which reflect the same differentiation in REBT theory. Thus, it does not trouble me to use the terms 'facilitative anxiety' and 'debilitative anxiety' instead of 'concern' and 'anxiety' with one client and 'helpful guilt' and 'unhelpful guilt' instead of 'constructive sorrow' and 'guilt' with another, as long as we both understand the distinctions we are making and they are consistent with REBT theory. Therapeutic alliance theory argues that if therapeutic change is to be enhanced you and your client need to speak the same language.

> **Key point**
>
> *Ensure that you and your clients develop a common language when discussing and implementing important principles of REBT.*

9 Maintain a goal-directed stance in therapy

REBT is one of the cognitive–behavioural therapies and as such is sensitive to the importance of identifying and working with client goals. However, working with client goals is more complex than may appear at first sight. For example, the goals that clients set may reflect the level of their psychological disturbance and if you take these goals at face value, you may unwittingly be encouraging clients to work towards self-defeating ends. This explains why Albert Ellis prefers to help clients to overcome their disturbances before helping them to achieve their goals.

Clients' goals are not static and continually change. As such you need to monitor them continually so that you and your client can obtain an accurate 'read out' of the client's goals at any point in the therapeutic process (see Point 44). As this can be quite complicated, I employ in individual therapy a concept derived from rational emotive behavioural marital therapy.

Rational emotive behavioural marital therapists distinguish between two different phases of therapy. Initially, they help members of a couple to overcome their emotional disturbances about their relationship, before tackling their dissatisfactions about the relationship. I find it helpful to explain to individual clients that we need to help them overcome their disturbance about events before we can help them to change their environment and work towards greater self-fulfilment. This distinction will help you and your clients to be clear concerning whether you are working to overcome a disturbance goal or working to maximise a self-fulfilment goal. I have heard many REBT sessions founder because it is clear to me as supervisor that the therapist is working on overcoming a disturbance goal which the client is resisting because she wishes either to change her environment or to work towards a self-fulfilment goal. If you and your client are working towards different goals the therapeutic alliance will be threatened.

Albert Ellis is quite critical of therapists who encourage clients to set goals for particular therapy sessions and I agree with him on this point. He argues that therapists who encourage clients to set goals for particular sessions may foist goals on their clients which they may not in fact have. As a consequence, clients may become discouraged if they do not achieve these 'false' session goals.

Over the years, I have seen many clients who have failed in one of the analytic therapies. One of the major reasons why they seek my help is that they want a more goal-directed approach to therapy. They particularly complain about the aimlessness of their previous therapy. Thus, it is important not to underestimate the importance that achieving goals is likely to have for most, if not all, clients.

> **Key point**
>
> *Help your clients to set realistic goals at different stages of the process of REBT and monitor these goals throughout therapy.*

10 Elicit your clients' commitment to effect change

While encouraging your clients to establish what their problems are and what they hope to gain from therapy is very important, it is just as important for you to elicit their commitment to effect change. This point combines the principle of taking a goal-directed stance in therapy with the principle of encouraging your clients to take responsibility for their own change. Encouraging your clients to make a commitment to effect change involves discussing with them what they are prepared to do to achieve their goals, and what sacrifices they are prepared to make. It may be a truism that there is no gain without pain, but it is invariably true.

Discussing with clients what they are prepared to do in order to achieve their goals and what this might involve is, in my opinion, tremendously important. REBT is unique as a therapeutic system for stressing the roles that low frustration tolerance and discomfort disturbance play in client problems and in preventing them from achieving their goals. However, it is also true that your clients are more likely to put up with such discomfort if they see clearly that it is part of what is going to make change possible. Thus, a central part of gaining your clients' commitment to effect change is to help them become aware of the fact that change almost invariably involves some kind of discomfort. If they choose to experience that discomfort for the purpose of achieving these goals, then they increase the likelihood that they will engage in the change-producing tasks that they need to carry out in order to achieve their goals. If you discuss this issue with them, then you will help them to commit themselves to the arduous business of personal change.

> **Key point**
>
> *Help your clients to commit themselves to personal change and discuss with them the necessity of tolerating discomfort in the change process.*

11 Strive for philosophical change, but be prepared to compromise

As an REBT therapist, you will know that striving for philosophical change with clients means helping them to surrender their irrational beliefs and adhere to a set of rational beliefs. This involves helping clients to: (1) dispute their musts, while adhering to and actualising their preferences; (2) give up their awfulising, while encouraging them to acknowledge that it is bad when certain obstacles to their goals exist; (3) tolerate what they believe they cannot tolerate; and (4) accept themselves and other people as unratable, complex, ongoing, ever-changing, fallible human beings rather than as equivalent to single cell amoeba which can be given a single rating. However, as I noted in *Current Issues in Rational–Emotive Therapy* (Dryden, 1987), there are other types of psychological change. For example, there is inferential change where you help clients to change their inferences and interpretations of a situation. There is behavioural change which involves helping clients to change their behaviour, and there is environmental change which involves encouraging clients to change the negative activating events in their lives.

REBT theory advocates that you are best placed to help clients make environmental changes after you have helped them achieve a fair measure of philosophical change. The problem is that clients frequently have different ideas and are unwilling or unable to achieve a minimal level of philosophical change which would enable them to work towards the other types of change, free from the effects of emotional disturbance. Thus, you need to be flexible and prepared to compromise on your preferred goal of effecting philosophical change. You need to realise that certain clients may be able to effect philosophical change *after* they have effected inferential, behavioural or environmental changes. Above all, you need to avoid working inflexibly towards philosophical change when your client is stubbornly resisting you on this point. Here, as elsewhere, therapeutic alliance considerations need to be balanced against the therapeutic ideals of REBT.

> **Key point**
>
> *Work towards goals which are as philosophical in nature as your clients are prepared to accept and realise that working with less ideal goals (such as inferential, behavioural or environmental change) may be preferable to losing clients by persisting with philosophical change.*

12 Engage clients in the most productive therapeutic arena

Psychotherapy can occur in different interpersonal contexts – individual, couple, family, and group therapy, as well as within a larger therapeutic community; I call these contexts therapeutic arenas (Dryden, 1984). In my experience, different clients thrive in different therapeutic arenas and I suggest that you ask yourself 'which therapeutic arena is most productive for my client at this point in the therapeutic process?'. While there are no hard and fast rules here, it seems sensible to outline for clients the different therapeutic arenas and their advantages and disadvantages and then help them to make a choice. If clients are given a choice and are then provided with an intervention that is in line with their choice, this is more effective than offering them an intervention that they have not chosen. Having said that, it is important to consider the exceptions to the view that 'the customer is always right'.

Let me now outline some of the advantages and disadvantages of each therapeutic arena from the perspective of REBT. Individual therapy is frequently the arena of choice at the outset for most clients who have intrapersonal difficulties and particularly those who would find exploring these difficulties in the context of group therapy overly threatening. Individual therapy, particularly with a therapist who is seen as understanding and trustworthy, enables such clients to reveal aspects of their experience which they might not reveal in other therapeutic arenas. This arena is particularly indicated where depth of client disclosure is a central part of the productive therapeutic process. However, some clients may have had too much individual therapy and need the challenge of working within a group context. Individual therapy may also be contraindicated for clients who cannot stand back and reflect on their transferential responses to their therapists.

Couple therapy is obviously indicated where the client's presenting problem is centrally rooted in the dynamics of a significant relationship. Here the challenge is to encourage the partner to come into couple therapy. Couple therapy is also useful when a significant other can be used as a therapeutic aide or where you wish to disarm the negative influence of a client's partner. Where marital problems are the focus of concern, conjoint couple therapy is indicated unless both partners disturb themselves about their problems in the presence of the other. In this case, you may need to see each person individually to help them overcome their disturbance before returning to conjoint work when marital dissatisfaction issues can be addressed.

Family therapy is the arena of choice where the presenting client problem is intimately connected to relationships within the family or where the presenting client is a child or early adolescent. Whether you can see the family as a unit depends upon: (1) your skill as an REBT family therapist; (2) the extent to which the family members disturb themselves about each other's presence; and (3) the extent to which the family denies problems when meeting as a total unit. Smaller units within the family may need to be seen before the family is seen as a whole.

As noted earlier, group therapy is indicated where a client has had considerable individual therapy previously, without deriving much benefit from it, and when the client's problems are rooted in general relationship difficulties with large numbers of people rather than with named significant others. Group therapy is also indicated when it is helpful for clients to learn that other people have similar difficulties and when they can experience themselves as being helpful to other people. Pragmatically, of course, it is often cheaper than individual therapy! Group therapy is not indicated, however, when your clients cannot 'share' you with other people, when they are extremely socially anxious and cannot concentrate in large groups of people and when they are unhelpfully manipulative or tend to monopolise the therapeutic process.

> **Key point**
>
> *Learn the strengths and weaknesses of different therapeutic arenas and engage your clients in the arena that is most productive for them.*

Part II

Educational Issues

13 Suggest that clients record and review their counselling sessions

As I noted in the first section of this book and as I will highlight here, REBT is an educational approach to psychotherapy. Thus your therapeutic endeavours can be seen as akin to those of an educator and the tasks of your clients as equivalent to those of students or learners. You therefore need to bear in mind various important educational principles in the way you conduct REBT.

One important point is that clients can become very preoccupied when they discuss their problems. They can become preoccupied with their past experiences or get caught up in their emotions as they experience them in the therapy room. They may then frequently fail to pay attention to what you are saying as their therapist and they may not appreciate the points that they are making to you. It is therefore often helpful for them to listen to therapy sessions later if they are to gain full benefit from them. So encourage your clients to make tape-recordings of therapy sessions for later review; it is often easier for clients to give permission for therapists to tape-record therapy sessions if they themselves are also allowed to make recordings. This puts into practice the principle of parity that REBT therapists hold dear.

A main advantage of clients tape-recording their sessions is that such recordings provide them with the opportunity to hear themselves express irrational beliefs that they may have denied having. Tape-recordings also give clients an opportunity to hear and appreciate, perhaps more fully than they did during therapy sessions, the points that you, as their therapist, were making to them. As one of my clients once said, 'whilst I was listening to you in the session my mind was preoccupied with what I was saying. However, when I listened to the tape afterwards, the full force of your arguments became crystal clear to me'. Also when clients listen to a recording of a therapy session they are often in a better frame of mind than when they are talking about their problems in the session. During the session they may be too disturbed or too distracted to benefit fully as the quote from my client amply demonstrates. Additionally, I have found that when clients listen to tapes of their therapy sessions, they initially often hold their therapist's voice in their mind when learning to dispute their irrational beliefs. Although you will want to wean them from this practice and encourage them to use their own voice later in therapy, as an initial strategy, tape-recording can facilitate the disputing process in this respect.

As with any therapeutic intervention, there are drawbacks with encouraging clients to listen to recordings of their therapy sessions. A small minority of clients, for example, may disturb themselves about the sound of their voice. If this happens, you might trying encouraging them to use REBT while listening to their voice, but in my experience this does not work, at least initially. Whenever your clients become overly preoccupied with how they sound or how they may have come across to you in the session, to the extent that they do not learn from listening to the session recording, it may be helpful to suggest to them that they stop recording the sessions, at least temporarily, and perhaps make notes during the therapy session.

Another drawback to taping REBT sessions is that some of your clients may come to overly rely on the tapes, so that they become passive rather than active learners. A sign that this is happening is when your client reports that he turns to the tape whenever he becomes upset, rather than using the tape to stimulate his own learning so that he can identify, challenge and change his irrational beliefs for himself when he becomes upset. Under these conditions, the tape becomes a crutch rather than a prompt. This may not be such a problem if you can identify and deal with it early on, but it can constitute an obstacle to the client becoming his own counsellor if he steadfastly uses the tape as a crutch. However, if the choice is between having your client listen to the tape in passive mode and not learning anything at all from therapy sessions, then I would still advocate the use of tape recordings.

> **Key point**
>
> *Encourage your clients to record and review therapy sessions as a way of facilitating their learning of rational principles.*

14 Educate clients in the model and process of REBT and help them understand your respective roles within that process

One of the most robust findings in the field of psychotherapy is the beneficial effect that anticipatory socialisation practices have on the process and outcome of therapy. When you prepare your clients to understand REBT and the roles that you and they have to play in the process, they will make more effective use of therapy. Such preparation can be done before clients come to therapy or early in the therapeutic process. In fact, if you do it before therapy starts you enable your prospective clients to make an informed decision about whether REBT is the therapy for them. If you do it after therapy has begun, choose a time which does not interfere with your clients discussing their problems! You might agree to use a portion of an opening session to describe REBT and discuss this with your client; you might even devote an entire session to this crucial point. Whichever method the two of you choose, it is important that you outline your tasks as a therapist and what will be expected of the client. Additionally, you may want your client to read something on REBT which makes clear your respective roles. Russ Grieger (1989) has prepared a client's guide to REBT which outlines in stepwise fashion what is expected of clients at different stages of the REBT therapeutic process. My experience of using this guide is that it is best given to clients bit by bit rather than in one chunk, because much of the guide depends on the client understanding the points previously introduced *and* experienced.

Different REBT therapists use anticipatory socialisation materials in different ways. My own practice is to explain the ABC model of REBT, the reason for my taking an active-directive approach, the importance of homework, and that the therapeutic process, like true love, does not always run smoothly! I do this in the first or second session whenever I can.

It is crucial to elicit client feedback on whatever material you present: first, it communicates to your client that you are taking her seriously as an active partner in the therapeutic process; second, the questions clients raise during feedback often provide useful clues to how you as a therapist may have to change your normal style to accommodate their idiosyncratic and healthy preferences. You may need to stress these changes when explaining your therapeutic style to a client. For example, if your client expresses concerns that an active-directive style could mean that she may not have much time to talk, bear this in mind and stress that you will give her an uninterrupted period to tell her story, something which in general REBT therapists tend not to do, but which I find to be quite helpful for a significant minority of clients.

An alternative way of discovering how you might need to change your usual therapeutic style is to ask your client to tell you how her ideal therapist would act. You may then incorporate some of these elements into your explanation of REBT and your role within it. In addition, you may usefully enquire what the client has found useful in the past about seeking help informally from other people or from formal helpers. Again you may incorporate helpful elements of past therapist behaviour in your explanation of your role as an REBT therapist, while carefully dealing with those aspects deemed helpful by the client which you would consider to be anti-therapeutic.

Key point

Teach clients the ABCs of REBT, and help them to understand your role as an REBT therapist and their role as an REBT client.

15 Explain what you are doing and why you are doing it

In the previous point, I stressed how important it is for you to make clear at the outset your own contribution to the therapeutic process and the reasons why you will often take an active-directive stance. What I want to stress here, however, concerns the ongoing process of psychotherapy. I believe that it is important for you to explain, at fairly regular intervals, not only what you are doing, but why you are doing it. If you can explain to your client the rationale for an intervention before you make it and if your client can indicate that it makes sense to her, this is a good way of gaining her co-operation. This is particularly useful if you plan to make interventions that may otherwise be perceived as strange or even aversive by your client. For example, if you plan to dispute your client's irrational beliefs in a vigorous, forceful manner, it is useful first to help her to understand why you plan to do this, so that your client sees that you are doing it in her interests and are not attacking her. This preparatory work is generally, in my experience, more helpful than explaining to the client after the fact why you have intervened in this way. I do not suggest that you do this in a compulsive way or indeed in a needy way. However, particularly when you plan to make unusual or potentially aversive interventions, helping clients to understand their purpose in advance constitutes, in my view, sound educational practice.

> **Key point**
>
> *Explain the purpose of your interventions to clients, particularly when these interventions are unusual and potentially aversive.*

16 Pay attention to clients' non-verbal and paraverbal behaviour

REBT sessions are quite verbal in nature and practitioners of other therapeutic schools are struck by the amount that the REBT therapist talks. However, this does not mean that good REBT therapists do not pay attention to their clients' non-verbal or paraverbal behaviour. Being sensitive to such client behaviour will help you gauge their reactions, particularly to any teaching points you might make.

In ordinary social conversation people often non-verbally or paraverbally indicate agreement or understanding, when in fact they may disagree with or not understand what is being communicated by the other person. This same principle also applies in the practice of REBT. You should not only look out for overt signs that your client disagrees with or does not understand what you are saying, but also be aware of signs that his subtle non-verbal and paraverbal cues contradict his stated agreement and understanding. Thus a client may state that he agrees with you but fidget quite a lot with his hands, which may be an indication of his true response.

Although I am not suggesting that you abandon REBT and become a gestalt therapist and encourage your clients to become aware of ongoing shifts in their non-verbal behaviour, I do recommend that you strive to understand the meaning behind the inconsistencies in your clients' responses, something that gestalt therapists are particularly sensitive to. When you identify such inconsistencies and draw these to your client's attention, you need to do this in a respectful way. In particular, you need to note your client's eye contact, hand movements, direction of eye gaze and tone of voice. For example, I have become adept at spotting the hidden 'but' in my clients' sentences by the tone of their voice and the way they move their body. I use such signs as cues to ask clients for a verbal account of their understanding of the points that I have made to them.

As I have said before, your main purpose is not just to teach rational principles to your clients but to encourage them to learn and apply these principles to their everyday lives. Thus, you need to check regularly what your clients are learning from what you are teaching them. Being sensitive to non-verbal and paraverbal clues to client understanding or lack of understanding is another part of this process.

> **Key point**
>
> *Pay attention to your clients' non-verbal and paraverbal behaviour. Such behaviour can provide important clues to your clients' true response to what you are saying.*

17 Teach and re-teach your clients the principle of emotional responsibility

One of the most fundamental principles that you can teach your clients is that of emotional responsibility. This principle is at the heart of the ABC model of emotional disturbance which states that it is *our* beliefs about the events in our lives that are centrally implicated in our emotional and behavioural responses to those events. This does not mean that these events do not contribute to our problems, but that they do not create or lie at the centre of our emotional experiences.

The principle that it is their beliefs that lie at the core of your clients' experiences and that they are responsible for these beliefs is a simple one which your clients may have enormous difficulty in grasping fully. I stress that they may have difficulty in fully grasping this principle because while they may intellectually understand it, being able to integrate it into their lives in a way that makes a fundamental difference to their lives is an entirely different matter. Thus, you need to keep returning to this principle and keep emphasising it, particularly when your clients indicate that events directly cause their emotional and behavioural responses.

I am not advocating that you bring this principle to your clients' attention *every* time they say something like 'he makes me upset' or 'she made me disturbed' etc. Far from it. Doing so will only serve as an irritant to your clients. However, you can usefully refer to the 'emotional responsibility' principle at important junctures in the therapeutic process since this will serve as a helpful reminder for clients to look at 'B–C' connections, rather than 'A–C' connections.

There are a number of ways in which you can encourage your clients to become more aware of the emotional responsibility principle. One is to suggest that they watch television and note the extent to which people use 'A–C' language. You can follow up on this by encouraging them to apply this exercise in real life. It may also be helpful for them to re-phrase people's language, so that they can get used to changing 'A–C' language to 'B–C' language. If, for example, a client hears somebody say 'He made me upset', she can change this to 'She made herself upset about what he said and this is how she did it'.

Encouraging your clients to look for the musts, awfulising, LFT and self/other downing in their and other people's thinking serves to reinforce the emotional responsibility principle. You can then help them see the connection between such beliefs and the ensuing emotional and behavioural responses.

I often find it helpful to work out a physical sign with clients which indicates to them that they are using 'A–C' language rather than 'B–C' language. For example, one sign that is particularly useful is when I pat myself on my head: this draws my clients' attention to the fact that they are neglecting the role that their brain plays in their emotional responses.

> **Key point**
>
> *Teach your clients the principle of emotional responsibility. Remind them of this principle without annoying them and encourage them to discover it for themselves both in their own experience and in the experiences of others.*

18 Teach the full distinction between rational beliefs and irrational beliefs

REBT is very clear about what constitutes an irrational belief. Generally speaking an irrational belief is self- and other-defeating, illogical and inconsistent with reality. It can take the form of a dogmatic must, awfulising, low frustration tolerance and self- and other- downing. An important part of helping your clients to challenge such beliefs is to teach them the distinction between these irrational beliefs and their rational alternatives. These rational beliefs are logical, consistent with reality and more productive with respect to self-enhancement and the development of healthy interpersonal relationships. Rational beliefs generally take the form of non-dogmatic desires, an evaluation of a negative event as being bad, high frustration tolerance and self- and other-acceptance.

Albert Ellis has often stated that clients easily escalate their rational beliefs to irrational beliefs. This means that if you merely teach your client that the rational alternative to a must is a preference (e.g. 'I would like to do well' rather than 'I must do well'), then the client may still tend to add an implicit must to his seemingly rational belief (e.g. 'I want to do well, therefore I have to do well'). Thus, it is important to teach clients the full distinction between a rational belief and an irrational belief. This means not only showing clients that a rational belief contains a preference statement, but also teaching them that it does not contain a must statement. Rather than show the client that an example of a rational belief is 'I would like to do well', teach her that the *full* rational belief is 'I would like to do well, *but I do not have to do so*'.

This also applies to the three irrational derivatives from the must. Thus, when helping a client to construct an anti-awfulising belief, rather than have her say: 'It is bad when I do not achieve what I want', teach her that the full rational belief is: 'It is bad when I do not achieve what I want, *but it is not the end of the world*'. Similarly, when dealing with a rational alternative to low frustration tolerance, it is important to stress that the full version of such as alternative is not 'I can stand it' but 'I can stand it, *even though I do not like it*'. Finally, a full rational alternative to a self-downing belief such as 'I am no good' is 'I am a fallible human being *even though I do more poorly than I would prefer to do*'.

Stating the full form of a rational belief explicitly, makes it less likely that your clients will implicitly or silently escalate seemingly rational beliefs into covert irrationalities.

> **Key point**
>
> *Teach your clients the full distinction between rational beliefs and irrational beliefs to help prevent them from implicitly escalating the former into the latter.*

19 Teach your clients to distinguish between healthy and unhealthy negative emotions

As far as I know, REBT is the only theoretical perspective in psychotherapy that keenly discriminates between what Ellis calls inappropriate and appropriate negative emotions (or what I prefer to call healthy and unhealthy negative emotions). As most of you will be aware, unhealthy negative emotions (e.g. anxiety, depression, guilt, anger) stem from irrational beliefs, while healthy negative emotions (e.g. concern, sadness, regret, annoyance) occur when people hold rational beliefs about adversities at A. As an REBT therapist, you will see those inappropriate or unhealthy negative emotions listed above as preventing your clients living emotionally healthy lives and therefore you will often target them for change. However, you need to be aware that your clients may have very different views on this issue and may interpret your emotional lexicon differently. For example, some clients consider anxiety useful in helping them achieve what they want; others regard guilt as necessary to protect them from doing bad things; yet others see anger as a constructive way of responding when others transgress their rules of living. Consequently, you need to spend time exploring with your clients the way they construe what you consider to be unhealthy negative emotions and correct any misconceptions like those listed above.

In addition, it is helpful to teach your clients the cognitive dynamics of healthy and unhealthy negative emotions. In doing so, you need to stress that these are clearly distinguished by the presence of irrational beliefs in the set of unhealthy negative emotions and the presence of rational beliefs in the set of healthy negative emotions.

If you fail to help your clients understand the distinction between healthy and unhealthy negative emotions and the cognitive correlates of each, you may threaten the therapeutic alliance by proceeding as if they do understand and agree with this distinction. Consider the effect on the therapeutic alliance of encouraging a client to (1) overcome his anxiety when he sees it as enhancing his performance; or (2) give up his guilt when he views guilt as a protection against wrongdoing. In the first case, you will be seen as discouraging achievement and in the second case, encouraging immorality.

These ruptures to the therapeutic alliance are less likely to occur if you help your clients to distinguish between healthy and unhealthy negative emotions and to see the value of working to minimise the latter in favour of the former when they face adversities at A.

> **Key point**
>
> *Teach your clients to distinguish between healthy and unhealthy negative emotions, help them understand the cognitive correlates of each type and encourage them to work towards feeling healthily negative in the face of life's adversities.*

20 Teach your clients the importance of dealing with emotional disturbance before they learn new skills or change their environment

Your clients will often come to therapy experiencing dysfunctional emotions. Some will find it difficult to understand that before they can learn new skills or change aversive activating events they will need to change the irrational beliefs that are at the core of their disturbed emotions. Others will grasp this point but may forget it later in therapy. It is therefore important that you use a number of analogies to show your clients the continuing importance of working to change their irrational beliefs before working at other levels of change. However, you must be prepared to compromise with your clients on this point if they steadfastly resist working to change their irrational beliefs (see p. 16).

One of the best ways that I have found to communicate this point so that clients learn and apply it, is to show them that when they make themselves emotionally disturbed they give themselves an additional problem. Thus instead of just facing the aversive activating event (problem 1), they make themselves disturbed about this event (problem 2). Once they are emotionally disturbed about the negative event, trying to change this event or learning new skills to bring about change without first overcoming their emotional disturbance is like trying to walk uphill with a ball and chain around one's leg; the emotional disturbance keeps dragging you back. Having explained this to clients, all I need to do subsequently is draw a picture of a ball and chain to remind them of this point.

Another analogy that I have found useful is helping a client to see that when he is anxious, he is running around like a headless chicken. 'Do headless chickens make healthy decisions for themselves?' No, what the headless chicken needs to do is to find its head so that it can think things through more constructively rather than dash around in all directions hoping to find a solution. Do not give too many analogies at any one time and once a client has indicated that she finds a particular analogy useful, keep using it rather than using different analogies to make the same point.

> **Key point**
>
> *Use analogies to teach your clients the value of dealing with their emotional disturbance before they attempt to change their environment or learn new skills.*

21 Teach your clients the effect of irrational beliefs on their interpretations of activating events

In REBT theory, the relationship between activating events (including interpretations of these events), beliefs, emotions and behaviours is exceedingly complex. Albert Ellis (1991) has argued that people bring their irrational beliefs to the interpretations they make of activating events and I have found it very useful to teach clients this important point.

Generally, in REBT, when your client describes an activating event (A), you will ask her to assume that A is true even though it may be obviously distorted. You will then help the client to identify her irrational beliefs about this distorted interpretation of A and then proceed to encourage her to dispute these irrational beliefs. After this has been done, freed from the disturbing effects of these irrational beliefs, your client can then challenge her inferential distortions of A.

Sometimes, however, if you encourage your client to assume that A is true then it may be extremely difficult to encourage her to challenge and change her irrational beliefs. For example, in panic disorder, a client often misinterprets the nature of her anxiety symptoms and may conclude that this means she is going to die. Although it is theoretically possible for you to encourage this client to assume temporarily that this is true and try to help her to identify and change her irrational beliefs about dying, on the few occasions that I have encouraged clients to do this, the results have been uniformly unproductive. A more productive strategy in such circumstances is for you to teach your client that when she holds irrational beliefs and brings these beliefs to events, then such beliefs will lead her to make distorted interpretations about the activating event. Indeed, such irrational beliefs and interpretations of A are often chained together and at the end of the chain, grossly distorted interpretations of A are produced such as 'I am going to die' (Dryden, 1989a).

In teaching clients about the effects of irrational beliefs on interpretations of A, I describe several experiments that I have done with some of my students on this very issue. In one experiment (Dryden, Ferguson and McTeague, 1989), we asked one group of subjects to imagine that they held the following irrational belief about spiders: 'I absolutely must not see a spider and it would be terrible if I did' and another group was asked to hold the following rational belief: 'I would much prefer not to see a spider, but there is no reason why I must not see a spider. It would be bad if I did see a spider but not terrible'. Both groups of subjects were asked to imagine that they were about to enter a room which had at least one spider in it. They were then asked a number of questions about the environment which they were about to enter, e.g. How many spiders are there in the room? How large are the spiders? Are the spiders moving randomly in the room, towards you or away from you? All these questions are focused on interpretative aspects of the A. The results of this experiment showed that when subjects held an irrational belief about spiders, this belief led them to make far more distorted interpretations of their environment than when they held a rational belief about spiders.

In addition, I often teach my clients that irrational beliefs and interpretations of A can interact with one another in a spiralling fashion (Dryden, 1989a). Thus, a client who brings an irrational belief about anxiety, for example, to a situation in which she starts to become anxious will then tend to make a distorted interpretation of A. She then brings a further irrational belief to this distorted interpretation with the result that she makes an even more distorted interpretation. The client then brings yet another irrational belief to this second distorted interpretation with the consequence that a third, even more distorted interpretation of A is made. This process can occur very quickly and implicitly, with the end result that the client can make an extremely distorted interpretation of A, about which she finds it extraordinarily difficult to think rationally. Teaching clients about the spiralling effect that irrational beliefs have on interpretations of A can help them understand what is going on in a situation where they are only aware of the last grossly distorted interpretation of A in the chain.

As well as teaching your client about this process, you can encourage him to focus on the beginning of such an episode and dispute his irrational beliefs about a mildly distorted interpretation of A. If you are successful, the spiralling process of interacting irrational beliefs and ever increasing distorted interpretations of A is brought under control.

> **Key point**
>
> *Rather than encouraging your clients to assume that grossly distorted interpretations of A are true, help them to understand how irrational beliefs produce ever increasing distorted interpretations in a spiralling process where A's and irrational beliefs interact.*

22 Teach your clients the difference between acceptance and resignation

In REBT theory acceptance has a particular meaning: it means an acknowledgement that a situation exists and it exists because all the conditions necessary for the situation to exist are in place. Acceptance does not preclude disliking the situation if it is aversive. In helping clients to accept aversive events, it is important for you to help them to give up their demands that such events must not exist and to surrender the magical idea that the conditions which were in place for the events to occur absolutely should not have existed. In short, the client is encouraged to acknowledge that reality should (empirically) be reality.

I have found it very important to explain precisely what is meant by acceptance to discourage clients from bringing their own meaning of this term to our therapeutic discussion. Frequently, your clients will confuse 'acceptance' with 'resignation' and will, if you are not careful, respond to you encouraging them to accept that an aversive situation exists as if you were encouraging them to resign themselves to the situation, i.e. they may imply that nothing can be done about this situation. Of course, nothing could be further from the truth. You need to explain to your clients that just because they accept that a situation exists and that a set of conditions is in place for this situation to exist, does not preclude them, in any way, from attempting to change the situation by modifying those extant conditions. If those conditions cannot be changed, then you need to encourage your client to accept this grim reality.

Acceptance, as defined here, is often a healthy prerequisite for adaptive behaviour, the purpose of which is to modify the existing aversive event and its extant preconditions. If your clients try to change situations when they are disturbed or demandingly non-acceptant of these situations, then their behaviour is likely to be maladaptive and therefore less successful. If demanding non-acceptance promotes maladaptive behaviour then resignation discourages clients from taking productive action. If they are resigned to a situation, then there is no motivation to change it.

A similar point arises when you encourage your clients to 'accept themselves as fallible human beings'. If you do not explain exactly what you mean by this phrase, your client may well misinterpret your meaning. When you encourage clients to accept themselves as fallible human beings, what you as REBT therapists are doing is urging them to refrain from making global ratings of their 'selves'. If your clients are able to do this to a reasonable degree, they are free to focus on whatever aspects of themselves they do not like and can attempt to change these. Once again acceptance (in this case self-acceptance) is often a prerequisite for adaptive action. However, if you are not careful, your clients may take away from discussions of self-acceptance the view that you have been urging them to *resign* themselves to the fact that there is nothing they can do to change an aspect of themselves that they do not like. Even if your clients do not bring up the resignation criticism of the concept of acceptance, it is productive for you to introduce this subject yourself, to emphasise the fact that you are *discouraging* resignation and *encouraging* healthy acceptance as a precursor for productive change.

> **Key point**
>
> *Teach your clients what the term acceptance means in REBT theory. In particular, help them to distinguish between acceptance, demanding non-acceptance and resignation.*

23 Teach relapse prevention

Relapse prevention is a term which originated in work with the addictions to highlight the fact that relapse often occurs and that a concerted effort to help clients prevent relapse is frequently necessary. A major part of relapse prevention involves helping clients to become aware of a variety of vulnerability factors. These client vulnerability factors can occur in their external and internal environment. Internal vulnerability factors include their styles of thinking, behaviour patterns and emotional responses, all of which serve as invitations to drink.

As you will know well, the course of therapy rarely runs smoothly and your clients will frequently take two steps forward and one step back and even one step forward and two steps back! When these setbacks are small and when they occur in the context of general client progress, they are best described as lapses. However, when a client experiences a significant setback this is perhaps better described as a relapse. In rational emotive behavioural relapse prevention, you ask your client to take each problem on her problem list and identify the set of internal and external circumstances in which she may experience a relapse. Help her as specifically as you can to identify relapse-triggering activating events, and the irrational beliefs she holds about such events. In particular, help her to identify any vulnerable feelings which may discourage her from using REBT techniques.

Then, encourage her to imagine that she is experiencing such a vulnerable feeling or entering into a situation in which she may be vulnerable to relapse and ask her to use her rational thinking skills to prevent the situation leading to relapse. She may do this by using imagery techniques or self-help forms. In fact, she can use any of the numerous REBT change techniques at this point. After she has successfully coped with this vulnerability factor in imagination, she is then encouraged to seek it out in reality so that she can gain experience of using her developing rational thinking skills in vivo. While doing this, it is particularly useful for you to bear in mind the points I made in the 'challenging but not overwhelming' point (see Point 6).

It is particularly important for you to encourage your client to accept herself if she fails to use her rational thinking skills in real-life vulnerable situations and experiences a relapse. Part of relapse prevention includes helping your client to think rationally about relapses and so get back on track having accepted herself for her relapse. When clients think rationally about relapse they can more easily learn from the experience than when they think irrationally about it.

> **Key point**
>
> *Teach your clients that they need to work to identify internal and external triggers to potential relapse. Help them to prevent such relapse by encouraging them to expose themselves to these triggers in imagery and in vivo. Doing so will show them that they can apply their rational coping skills should they encounter their vulnerability factors.*

Education issues

24 Teach your clients the principles of REBT self-therapy

One of the ultimate goals of REBT is to encourage clients to serve as their own counsellors after formal therapy has come to an end. While you will be gratified when your clients have made therapeutic gains at the end of therapy, you will not consider that you have fully done your job unless you have taught them a self-change methodology. Unless your clients can apply what they have learnt in therapy to their lives at their own prompting, then whatever gains they may have achieved from therapy will probably not be maintained in the long run. Unless your clients have internalised a set of self-helping strategies and techniques, then they may well fail to deal with any new aversive activating events that they might encounter.

Thus, your central task as an REBT therapist is to: (1) introduce the concept of self-help into therapy and (2) systematically help your clients to acquire REBT self-help skills. You can best do this in a structured way. Thus, you can formally and deliberately teach your clients such REBT skills as: (1) using a variety of self-help forms; (2) identifying clinically relevant aspects of negative activating events; (3) discriminating keenly between their rational beliefs and their irrational beliefs; and (4) challenging and changing in a vigorous manner their irrational beliefs. You can also teach them the large number of emotive and behavioural techniques which will help them to weaken their irrational beliefs and strengthen their rational beliefs.

Once you have taught your clients these skills in a structured and deliberate way, then you need to encourage them to use the skills on their own. You can serve as their consultant while they do this, providing them with useful feedback on any problems they may experience in this phase of therapy. It is important that you give your clients an opportunity to serve as their own therapist as early in the process as is clinically indicated. When this is handled successfully, you can reduce your active input into the therapeutic process while encouraging your clients to become more active in applying the skills they have learnt during therapy to their own lives.

However, do not expect that all of your clients will be able to become their own therapist. Some of them may be so handicapped that they may not find it possible to serve as their own therapist for any extended period of time. In such cases you will need to use your clinical commonsense and not expect too much. If you have unrealistic expectations of such clients you may unwittingly discourage them from using the limited self-help abilities that they do possess.

Key point

As soon as you can, introduce the concept of self-help into REBT and teach your clients the skills of REBT self-help therapy in a structured and deliberate manner. Realise that clients differ markedly in their ability to act as their own therapist. Consequently, use your clinical commonsense and develop realistic expectations concerning the extent to which each of your clients can serve as their own therapist.

Part III

Technical Issues

25 Be organised and structured in therapy sessions

REBT is a structured approach to psychotherapy. Thus, if you are to practise REBT effectively you will need to organise and structure your therapy sessions with your clients. In order to sustain the therapeutic alliance you should provide your clients with a rationale for the use of structure in REBT. In this rationale, you should stress that you will vary the amount of structure at different points in the therapeutic process and that this can be discussed with the client in the reflection process.

In 1981, I trained in cognitive therapy at the Center for Cognitive Therapy in Philadelphia. I learned from cognitive therapists the power of *agenda-setting* to provide a helpful structure at the outset of therapy sessions. Setting an agenda with your clients is a useful way of ensuring that important items that you both wish to address are covered in a therapy session or, if they are not, they may be put on the agenda for the following session. Typical items that you can put on an agenda include: (1) homework assignments from the previous session; (2) issues that your client wishes to address at the beginning of therapy – this will normally be what the client has been preoccupied with or disturbed about since the previous week; (3) the client's reactions to any unfinished business from the previous session; and (4) at the end of a session, your client's reactions to the work that you have done. In addition you may include, as therapist, any issues that you deem important to discuss. Agenda items should be prioritised so that efficient and effective use can be made of therapeutic time.

Albert Ellis's (1989) view of agenda-setting is that it may foster unhelpful consumerism and may, in fact, lead to avoidance of core problems in that it encourages clients with LFT to focus on issues that are less threatening for them to address. While this danger certainly exists, if you negotiate agenda-setting with your client rather than accepting uncritically what she wishes to cover, it will be minimised. In particular, look for items that your client has put on her problem list or for problems that she has listed on intake questionnaires that she avoids including in her agenda items. Place these issues on the agenda at some point during the therapeutic process and discuss with your client the reasons for their omission. So far from being an overly consumeristic activity, agenda-setting, if used responsibly, can be an important way of ensuring that therapy sessions are well organised and well structured.

Agreeing an agenda for a therapy session gives both you and your client a way of evaluating the introduction of new material into the session. If you use agenda-setting flexibly then you can discuss with your client whether a new issue is important enough for the agenda to be modified, or of minor importance. If the latter, then the previously agreed agenda needs to be retained and the new item can be tabled for discussion later in therapy. I hope it is clear, then, that agenda-setting is an additional way of strengthening the working alliance between you and your client in REBT.

I mentioned earlier that it is important to vary session structure. For example, there may well be times when your client is disturbed about a new issue in his life and at these times you may profitably loosen the structure of the session to enable the client to explore his feelings and reactions to this issue in an open-ended manner. If you allow the client to do this, you can always tighten the structure later to help him to identify more formally his irrational beliefs about this activating event.

You also need to vary session structure according to clients' different personality styles. You will find it particularly important to maintain a tight structure when working with clients who have a histrionic personality organisation. Doing so will serve as a model for them as you help them begin to structure and organise their own experiences without uncontrolled hysterical displays. However, for clients with obsessive-compulsive personality organisation, you will need to be less structured to encourage them to relax their own tightly organised controls. However, you will need to do this gradually as they will be unable to tolerate easily too little structure too soon in the therapeutic process.

> **Key point**
>
> *Be structured in the conduct of therapy sessions by using agenda-setting and other structuring methods. Be prepared to vary your use of structure with different clients at different points in the therapeutic process.*

26 Obtain sufficient information to help you carry out your therapeutic tasks

In my experience, REBT therapists vary considerably concerning how much information they obtain from their clients during the therapeutic process. Some REBT therapists prefer to follow the medical or psychiatric practice of conducting a fairly rigorous assessment at the outset of therapy. In the process they gain a lot of information, much of which may prove to be redundant, in that it is not used during therapy. Other REBT therapists do not carry out a structured assessment at the beginning of therapy, preferring to start by teaching clients the ABCs of REBT and to use this framework to obtain relevant information on clients. Such therapists assess as they continue therapy. Over the years I have experimented with both types of approach to information gathering and consider that both have their strengths and weaknesses.

The strength of carrying out comprehensive formal assessment at the outset, where an enormous amount of information on clients is gathered, is that you can learn to understand your clients from a holistic framework and can build up a picture of how their problems may relate to one another. However, even though you may provide a plausible rationale for such an approach, many clients may become impatient with a long and drawn-out assessment phase, particularly those who consider therapy to be a relatively brief intervention. The danger here is that some clients may well drop out of therapy before it has, in effect, begun, because they become frustrated that you are not addressing their concerns more quickly.

The problem of not carrying out a detailed assessment at the beginning is that you may overlook important information that your client may not reveal unless you specifically ask for it. On two memorable occasions, I learned fairly late in therapy that a client had a drinking problem. In response to my questions concerning why they did not inform me of this, they said 'Because you never asked!' (Dryden, 1992).

I now recommend a middle ground position, although I will carry out a fairly detailed assessment if the case is likely to be complex and I will also begin therapy quite quickly if, for example, my client has limited time. Thus, several of my past clients have come from out of town and wanted only to spend two or three sessions in therapy with me. Here, I get down to work straightaway and avoid carrying out a lengthy assessment.

I do recommend that you use a structured life history questionnaire such as Lazarus and Lazarus's (1991) *Multimodal Life History Inventory*, which enables you to gain a fairly comprehensive understanding of your client without utilising session time for this purpose. Of course, you need to follow up on any client responses on the questionnaire that need exploring and you need to investigate any important omissions. In general, however, this approach provides a way of understanding your clients in their historical and interpersonal contexts in a time-efficient manner.

When clients begin to address their problems in REBT there are two information gathering pitfalls to avoid. First, you need to avoid spending too much time gathering information that is not central to an understanding of the ABC of the client's problem. In particular, avoid the temptation of gaining too much unnecessary information about the client's A. Your clients are generally quite eager to talk expansively and irrelevantly about the A's in their lives and you may reinforce this tendency if you are not careful. Second, if you do not spend some time understanding the context in which a particular A occurs, then you may miss important, relevant information. For example, if your client is angry at her father's unreasonable behaviour it makes a difference to the work that you will do on this particular problem if her father has a psychiatric problem or has just learned that his own mother has died. Therefore, you need to guard against jumping in too quickly, and bypassing important information about the client's A.

> **Key point**
>
> *Gain sufficient information to enable you to practise REBT effectively. Be flexible in your information-gathering strategies. Sometimes, you will need to carry out a comprehensive structured assessment, while at other times you will need to use the ABC framework immediately. Use questionnaires as a time-efficient means of gathering relevant information about your clients.*

27 Keep on track

Ordinary social conversation between two people can range quite widely over a variety of issues. For example, you may meet a friend unexpectedly whom you have not seen for a while and you may begin your conversation by enquiring about each other's health. This might lead you to comment on the fact that you went to your doctor recently and that your family physician does not have a waiting list. Your friend might take up the issue of waiting lists and then tell you that he has applied to a local college, but has been placed on the waiting list. You may then ask how he hopes this course will help his career to which he may respond by telling you about his concern for his job due to the economic recession. You may then tell him about your financial problems which may lead to a discussion about the British economy. You may then go on to discussing politicians who cannot be trusted which may in turn lead to a conversation of the meaning of trust, etc.

Thus, much social interaction permits tangential changes in the direction of conversation. Indeed such changes grease the wheels of interpersonal relationships. So, when clients come to REBT, they bring with them a long history of interacting with people in a tangential manner. This tendency may be exacerbated if your clients have been in the type of psychotherapy which encourages tangential talk. Thus clients who have been in non-directive or psychoanalytic therapy may have been encouraged to explore their concerns in an open, unstructured manner. These approaches reinforce tangential talking. Consequently, you may have to educate your clients about the importance of keeping

Technical issues

on track when discussing their problems and tell them that, from time to time, you may interrupt them politely in order to keep them focused on their problems. You need to explain that tangential talk is a natural human tendency and ask their permission to interrupt them if you consider that they are going off the point. Asking for permission is less disruptive to the therapeutic alliance than interrupting clients without such an explanation and without gaining permission.

I mentioned on pp. 39–40 that keeping to an agenda is important, but that the agenda needs to be dealt with flexibly so that new information can be evaluated to determine whether its introduction will enhance the therapeutic process or de-rail it. Such evaluation is also salient here. For example, a client may introduce material that he believes is important, particularly when he begins to make associations between events. Thus, your client may be discussing a problem about his boss at work and then suddenly say that this problem reminds him of how he used to act towards his father. Since therapy involves you in a series of choice points, it is important that you have some way of knowing whether this new information enhances or derails the therapeutic process. If you think that the new issue is important then you may permit the change in tack. Unfortunately, there are few hard and fast rules that can be followed here, since the importance of new information has to be judged according to the dynamics of a particular case. So, evaluate the importance of the new material with your client and decide whether you need to change tack or keep to the original issue. If you have established the reflection process (see p. 12) then, at least, you will have a forum for such discussion.

Some therapists believe that the more uncomfortable a client is about a particular issue, the closer you may be getting to the real core of her problem and thus the more tangential the client is likely to be, given her need to change the topic of conversation. This certainly needs to be borne in mind and you need to have a detailed understanding of typical ways in which clients defend themselves against painful experience. You can then judge whether or not a client is employing such a mechanism in order to deflect you from a painful core issue. Another way you can evaluate the importance of newly introduced material is to ask your client how the new information is related to her problems at hand and whether it is central, important but not central, or unimportant. If you teach clients to use such categories to evaluate such information, this is another helpful way of keeping therapy on track.

> **Key point**
> *Realise that clients will often change the topic of conversation in therapy. Evaluate with the client the importance of the new information and decide whether to change tack or keep to the original issue.*

28 Choose the most suitable problem

When a client only brings one problem to therapy, then your life as therapist is made relatively simple, in that it is clear what you and your client need to work on. However, even in 'single problem' therapy the situation is still more complex than it may seem because your client may have a practical problem related to her emotional problem. She may also have a secondary emotional problem about her primary emotional problem. How do you and your client choose what is most suitable to tackle at a given point?

One rule is that you need to tackle emotional problems before practical problems. In order for your client to deal competently with a practical problem, she needs to be in a healthy frame of mind. Another guideline is that you often need to deal with secondary emotional problems before primary emotional problems, because it is difficult for your client to concentrate on dealing with one emotional problem if she is secondarily disturbed about that problem.

However, clients rarely come to therapy with only one problem; more commonly they have a myriad of problems each possibly complicated by the existence of a practical problem and a secondary emotional problem. The primary task that you and your client need to accomplish is to select and work on the client's most suitable and relevant problem.

In order to bring some order to this complexity, it is important that you and your client have a working understanding of the problems that the client wishes to address in therapy. Thus I recommend that you follow your cognitive therapy colleagues and develop with your client a problem list. This provides you both with an up-to-date picture of client problems to be discussed. Explain to your client the importance of this list and begin to compile it during the opening sessions of REBT. Then, as homework, encourage her to complete the list and to bring two copies to the following session, one for her to retain and one for you. Stress that you will need ready access to the list as you may need to add or delete items as you progress in therapy. Stress also that during therapy you may identify a small number of core irrational beliefs which may account for most of the problems on the client's list.

Having encouraged your client to develop a problem list, ask her to rank the problems in order of priority in which she wishes to deal with them. Explain to your client that she may wish to deal with problems that are perhaps less uncomfortable than others. This may not necessarily be productive so encourage your client to keep this point in mind while ranking the items. Once you have this list in prioritised order you can begin to work on a specific problem.

Once you have begun to work on a specific problem, remain with it until you have gone through the rational emotive behavioural treatment sequence (see Dryden, 1990a). As I will discuss later (see Point 33), you need to avoid working with different client problems in different sessions without achieving resolution on any problem. The risk of asking your client at the beginning of a session, what problem she would like to discuss in the session, is that she may focus on the most recent problematic activating event. If you deal with this, you may not complete the work you began in the previous session. If you use the rational emotive behavioural treatment sequence, it is important that you complete the sequence with a given problem before applying it to a second problem: remain with a problem once you and your client have started to work on it. There will, of course, be exceptions to this rule but by and large it is a good rule to follow.

In a workshop given in 1988, Raymond DiGiuseppe outlined the following order in which clients' problems need to be tackled, all other things being equal. He argued that problems of violence need to be dealt with first, because they constitute immediate threats to the well-being of the client and/or the client's significant others. Work and economic problems need to be dealt with next before sex and interpersonal problems, because in Ray's opinion, losing one's job is more serious than having a sex or interpersonal problem. Ray argues that clients are more able to live uncomfortably with their sex and relationship problems than they are with not having a job. I would agree with DiGiuseppe's analysis, although I would add that it is senseless for you to impose your own ideas on your clients if they have very different ideas. Here, as elsewhere, I would encourage you to work in a way that preserves the developing working alliance between you and your client.

Another issue that you need to consider here is whether you and your client should begin with a problem that is quite pervasive in the client's life and therefore quite difficult to solve, or with a problem that is less pervasive and that is more readily solved. If you begin with a client problem that may be quickly resolved, this may instill hope in your client that change is possible and may help to establish your credibility in the client's eyes. On the other hand, if your client is preoccupied with the more pervasive problem, then it is unlikely that she will achieve resolution on the less pervasive issue since her attention is elsewhere.

In conclusion, be flexible in deciding with clients which problem you are to tackle first. Gaining the client's commitment to work on a problem is perhaps the most important ingredient of all.

Key point

Consider various issues when deciding with your clients which problems to work on. Discuss these issues openly with your clients and gain their commitment to work on whichever problems you both consider most suitable.

29 Ask for specific examples of clients' problems

Clients make themselves disturbed in specific contexts. It is therefore important for you to encourage them to be specific in talking about their problems, and ask for specific examples. This will help you to conduct an accurate assessment of the ABCs of the problem. Encouraging your client to be specific about his problems will also help him to be emotionally involved in the discussion. If he talks about his problems in abstract terms, you will receive a general, intellectual and unemotional account. This will make it very difficult for you to conduct a meaningful assessment of his problems and make it harder for you to help him.

How can you help your client to be as specific as possible? First, you can encourage him to identify a recent example of his problem or a typical example of his problem. Make sure, though, that he chooses an episode where his feelings were fully engaged and which will help you to understand as clearly as you can what factors were involved in the problem.

If your client provides you with a relevant and specific example of his problem, then you can help him to identify the most relevant part of the A (see Point 32) as well as the precise emotions he experienced in the episode. If your client can identify clear relevant As and specific emotions, this will enable you to help him identify which specific irrational beliefs were at the core of his problem. This, in turn, encourages focused disputing of his irrational beliefs which will facilitate therapeutic change.

If your client routinely finds it difficult to identify specific examples of his problems, you will have to accept working with vague abstractions, if you are to help him at all. If this is so, then accept the grim fact that you may only be able to help him in a minimal way. However, do not give up, since helping someone to improve marginally is better than not helping him at all.

> **Key point**
>
> *Encourage your clients to be as specific as possible in discussing their problems. Doing so will help you to assess their problems accurately and will facilitate therapeutic change.*

30 Work a problem through

As mentioned in Point 28, it is important to persist at working on a problem once you and your client have targeted it for change (such a problem is known as a target problem). Several years ago, Ray DiGiuseppe and I formulated what is now called the rational emotive behavioural treatment sequence, in which we outlined 13 steps that you need to take if you are to deal with your client's target problem thoroughly (Dryden and DiGiuseppe, 1990). Unless you have good reason to do otherwise, encourage your client to remain focused on this problem and to work it through until she has reached coping criterion on it. This means that your client has had some practice at acting on her newly constructed rational belief in real-life situations and has gained some success at doing so. Thus, when your client introduces new material into the session, you need to evaluate this quite carefully and give only really important new material primacy over the current problem under discussion. Otherwise therapy will proceed in a way that is reminiscent of several half eaten meals.

There are, however, several situations that occur in therapy when it is justifiable for you and your client to switch your attention away from the target problem. The first concerns the development of a crisis in your client's life. When your client faces a new acute problem in her life, particularly involving suicidal ideation or violence, then it is important for you to deal with this problem without delay and persist in working with it until the client has met coping criterion. The only exception to this rule is with a client for whom every problem is a crisis. If this is the case, you need to model calmness and show her that she can work through the previously agreed target problem, even though the new problem has just appeared in her life.

Another indicator for switching from the target problem to a new problem is when your client becomes very disturbed in a session (this is her second problem) and cannot concentrate on the original problem. When this occurs, switch to the second problem and persist with it until coping criterion has been reached.

A third situation where you may preferably switch to a new problem is when a major new activating event occurs in the client's life such as a bereavement, job loss, or sudden illness. Failing to do so would be insensitive and counter-therapeutic. Here again you should switch and focus on this new adversity until the client reaches coping criterion.

The final indicator for switching away from work on a target problem is when it is clear that another problem has more pervasive negative effects on your client's life. For example, you may be working on a target anxiety problem when the client reveals a more pervasive problem of depression. If this occurs, switch and persist in working with the depression problem until again coping criterion has been reached.

> **Key point**
>
> *Once you have agreed target problems with your clients, work on these problems until they have reached coping criterion. Consider and implement the exceptions to this basic rule.*

31 Take care in your use of questions

As an REBT therapist, you will make liberal use of questions during the therapeutic process. You will use questions both to gain information about your client as you carry out a detailed assessment of his problems, and to encourage your client to identify, challenge and change his irrational beliefs. Since questions form such a central part in your therapeutic armamentarium, you need to use them with care and it is important for you to avoid the following errors when making use of questions.

Asking irrelevant questions

When using questions as part of gaining an overall understanding of your client, avoid asking irrelevant questions. In particular, avoid asking questions that arise out of your own curiosity about a client rather than help gain a full clinical understanding of that client and his problems. To ascertain the extent to which you may be asking irrelevant questions, tape-record a random selection of your therapy sessions and as you review them, ask yourself: 'Why did I ask that question?' 'Did I really need to know that information or did I ask just to satisfy my own curiosity?'

Asking vague questions

When you are assessing the ABCs of your client's problem, you need to ask questions which encourage the client to focus on specific aspects of the activating event and his disturbed feelings and behaviours. This will enable you more easily to identify his irrational beliefs. Your use of vague questions will generate vague answers and this will interfere with the assessment process.

Asking too many 'why' questions

'Why' questions may well encourage your client to become defensive in that he may experience your enquiry as criticism, or to speculate on

Technical issues

specious reasons for his behaviour, which may lead both of you up the garden path.

Bombarding your client with too many questions

This is a risk particularly in the disputing stage of therapy. Some REBT therapists that I have heard or supervised over the years sound like demented prosecution lawyers who just fire question after question at the client as if he is a hostile witness. This is rarely, if ever, productive. So when you ask questions, particularly while disputing the client's irrational beliefs, ensure that you do so with tact, sensitivity and in a way that enables your client to think about his answers.

Failing to evaluate your client's responses

When asking the client a question, make sure that you evaluate the answers that the client provides. I want to stress this because your client may fail to answer the question that you have asked or may answer a question that you did not ask. A good rule of thumb is this. When you ask a question that has a specific therapeutic purpose, evaluate your client's answer and if you consider that she has not answered your question, tactfully bring this to her attention and ask the question again.

Failing to provide ample opportunity for client responses

If you have asked your client a good question, give her the opportunity to answer it. REBT therapists with a philosophy of low frustration tolerance may well be too impatient to enable their clients to really think about questions that may be difficult to answer. Such therapists often answer their own questions – particularly in the disputing phase of a session.

For example, you might ask the question 'Where is the evidence that you have to do well?' Your client may not immediately reply, time might elapse and you may well find yourself answering the question for the client, 'There is no evidence that you have to do well, it is only desirable for you to do so.' Since one of your major goals as an REBT therapist is to encourage your client to think for herself, it is important to give her the opportunity to do so. Resist the temptation of answering your own questions!

Failing to alter your style of questioning

It is important that you ascertain whether or not your client readily responds to socratic questioning. Socratic questions are, of course, those which encourage clients to think for themselves and tend to be open ended. Some of your clients, however, will find it very difficult to answer socratic, open-ended questions and if you continue to use such questions, this will be both frustrating and countertherapeutic. If you find that a client does not respond well to socratic questions, alter your style of questioning and consider using forced choice questions. For example, instead of asking a client 'What do you think you were telling yourself to make yourself anxious?' you might ask, 'Were you thinking that you had to do well or that you would like to do well, but did not have to?'

Failing to make suitable use of open-ended and theory-derived questions

It is important that you distinguish between open-ended questions and theory-derived questions. An example of an open-ended question would be 'What were you telling yourself to make yourself anxious?' while a theory-derived question is one that is derived from REBT theory, e.g. 'What were you demanding of yourself to make yourself anxious?' Using too many open-ended questions with some of your clients is counter-productive because they may not have the patience to work out for themselves the distinction between preferences and demands, for example. If this is the case, give a brief didactic explanation of this distinction, and follow this up with theory-derived questions. However, with other clients who do have the facility to think clearly for themselves and prefer to be independent thinkers, open-ended questions may well be profitably employed in preference to theory-derived questions.

> **Key point**
>
> *Take care in the way you ask questions in REBT and learn which questioning errors to avoid.*

32 Take great care in assessing A

In REBT theory, A stands for an activating event. Initially this concept seems a simple one and yet it masks a great deal of complexity:

1. An activating event may form a small part of a larger environmental context in which your client finds herself and when she describes A to you she may talk about the larger context and not pinpoint the small component about which she was disturbed.

2. As noted by Wessler and Wessler (1980), As are frequently interpretations of what clients perceive. So, when your client says that she was giving a talk to a group of students and they were all bored with her presentation, she is clearly pointing not to an actual situation, but one that she has interpreted. As Bob Moore (1983) has emphasised, inferences are frequently chained together and when this occurs it is your task to help your client identify the most relevant aspect of the inferential chain, i.e. the inference that triggers the client's irrational beliefs which underpinned her distress.
3. We have the capacity to focus on different aspects of an activating event broadly at the same time. We evaluate those aspects in different ways and these evaluations (or irrational beliefs) lead to different disturbed feelings. Therefore, if you make the assumption that your client has only one feeling about an activating event you will grossly oversimplify your client's experience.
4. As discussed in Point 21, your client's interpretation of an activating event is frequently coloured by her irrational beliefs and when this is grossly exaggerated (e.g. 'I am going to die'), it is unwise to encourage her to assume that it is true, since it is unlikely that you will help her think rationally about such a tragedy.

Given the complexity of an activating event (A), it is very important that you take great care in assessing it. Keep in mind the following key questions as you do so.

1. Am I assessing the most clinically relevant part of the A, i.e. the one that triggered my client's irrational belief?
2. Am I choosing to work with an A about which my client can think rationally or do I need to explain the influence of her irrational beliefs on her inferences? If the latter, you need to help her identify a less negative A which occurs earlier in the inferential chain. You can then identify her irrational beliefs about this A and show her how these produce her grossly exaggerated inferences that occur later in the chain.

Another strategy that you can use to reduce the confusion which may arise from the complexity of A's, is to train your client to identify for herself the most relevant part of the A about which she was disturbed. Encourage her to ask herself: 'What was I most disturbed about in that situation?', or teach her inference chaining. When you train your client to identify the element of the A about which she was most disturbed, encourage her to identify her major disturbed emotion. Have her then review the episode in her mind and encourage her to use this feeling to locate the aspect of the situation that triggered her irrational belief. To the same end you can teach her to ask herself 'What was the worst thing that happened in this situation that I was disturbed about?' This is a very different question from, 'What was the worst thing that *could have* happened in this situation...?' At this point you are more interested in what your client was actually disturbed about than what she could have been disturbed about.

Training your client to use inference chaining is quite complex and in all probability only a minority of your clients will be able to do this effectively – this technique is difficult enough for REBT therapists to master effectively! When you do teach your client inference chaining, use the procedure outlined by Moore (1983) in his excellent step-by-step guide to this technique. Remember that the purpose of inference chaining is to identify the most clinically relevant part of your client's A and not necessarily to identify underlying core beliefs. Of course, it can be and has been used in this way, particularly by cognitive therapists (see Burns, 1980, for a discussion of the downward arrow technique).

Finally, after you have worked with a client for some time, you begin to gain an understanding of the types of A's about which she disturbs herself. You can, therefore, help your client to identify a theme in her disturbance and to use this theme as a guide to help her identify specific troublesome A's in her life. Thus, if your client has talked about several events in therapy that suggest that she disturbs herself about rejection, then you might encourage her to ask herself whether she considers that she has been rejected whenever she is upset in a social situation.

Later on in the therapeutic process, when it becomes clearer that your client has one or more core irrational beliefs about recurring themes at A, you can work at a more abstract level to help her identify and work with thematic A's. Do this later in the therapeutic process since, as I have argued elsewhere in this book, clients do not disturb themselves about general themes; rather they disturb themselves about specific events that may exemplify these themes.

> **Key point**
>
> *Realise that assessing A is more complex than it appears at first sight. Strive to find the most clinically relevant A in your clients' problems.*

33 Focus on core irrational beliefs

A core irrational belief is a belief which accounts for a significant proportion of your client's disturbance and which explains why your client upsets himself in a variety of different settings. A core irrational belief tends to be general rather than specific and can best be identified after you have worked with the client on identifying his specific irrational beliefs. An example of a core irrational belief might be: 'I must be in control in significant areas of my life. If I lose control, it would be awful and reveal something rotten about me.' Your client may express this core irrational belief in a specific form in a given specific environmental context. Thus, if your client has such a core irrational belief, he may be anxious about speaking in public because he fears that he may lose control of his fluency. He may also have difficulty forming close interpersonal relationships because he believes that he must have the upper hand and be in control of such relationships. Avoidant behaviour can also give a clue to the existence of a core irrational belief. Thus your client may tend to avoid situations which threaten his sense of control.

Some REBT therapists believe that it is important to devise a case formulation for each client, by which they mean working to develop an overall picture of a client's core irrational beliefs, showing how these may influence specific irrational beliefs, explain emotional, physiological and behavioural symptom patterns and how they may be implicated in the client's interpersonal relationships. What is important here is that you help your client not only to identify his core irrational beliefs, but also to understand the effect they have on his current life and the effect that they may continue to have on his life in the future if he does not change them. Thus, if your client has a core irrational belief about dependency, help her to see that holding this belief may lead her to construct her life so that she is always involved with a person even though that person may not be suitable for her. Also show her that she may construct her life so that she does not experience the discomfort of independence and this may explain why she does not take risks even though she keeps complaining about not fulfilling her potential.

Core irrational beliefs not only explain why your clients disturb themselves in a variety of settings, they also explain why they limit themselves and opt for short-term comfort rather than long-term gain. Thus, a client with a core irrational belief regarding dependency may seek out familiar situations in which she encourages other people to look after her because she experiences comfort in doing so, even though this behaviour interferes significantly with her long-range happiness.

In working with your client at the level of a core irrational belief, help her also to construct a core rational belief and to see how life could be different were she to believe and act on this more healthy core belief. Help your client also to take a realistic view of personal change. Not only help her to see the long-term advantages of changing core beliefs, but also encourage her to accept the short-term disadvantages of doing so, e.g. she will need to tolerate discomfort and a sense of unfamiliarity. As therapy proceeds, remind your client to look for a core irrational belief as well as her specific irrational beliefs in specific situations. Teach your client to ask herself such questions as 'Is this my dire need for control rearing its ugly head?' Helping your client to realise that she needs to dispute her core irrational belief repeatedly and in different contexts is particularly important, as is encouraging her to act in a way that is consistent with her newly constructed core rational belief and inconsistent with her old core irrational belief.

Finally, you need to help your client to generalise her core rational belief from one area of her life to other areas of her life that you may not have discussed in therapy. Part of this process also involves dealing with possible lapse and relapse. Since core irrational beliefs are more central in your client's belief system and have more pervasive effects, they are harder to change and this means that emotional and behavioural lapses and relapses are quite likely. Help your client to accept this grim reality and to employ the relapse prevention measures discussed on pp. 33–34.

> **Key point**
>
> *Realise that core irrational beliefs may underlie many of your clients' irrationalities. Focus on these core beliefs and help your clients to change them. Appreciate the difficulty of this task.*

34 Look for hidden irrational beliefs in elements of your clients' verbalisations and behaviours

In the early phase of REBT you will: (1) work with your client to identify his disturbing feelings and self-defeating behaviours; (2) teach him the ABCs of REBT; and (3) dispute his specific irrational beliefs. As discussed in the previous point, you will then help your client to identify, challenge and change his *core* irrational beliefs. Additionally, from the middle of therapy onwards, it is helpful to encourage your client to identify *subtle* irrational beliefs that may be present in his verbalisations and behaviour, but which may not be immediately related to disturbed feelings and behaviours at C. Doing this is important if you are to help your client make a thoroughgoing change in his irrational philosophies.

Clients may subtly hold on to their irrational beliefs, because they do not realise the impact that these have on a wide range of their verbalisations and behaviours. In the beginning phase of therapy, you need to be alert to the existence of hidden irrationalities implicit in your client's verbalisations and behaviour and you can utilise this material to help yourself form and test hypotheses about the nature of your client's explicit irrational beliefs. However, do not deal with these hidden irrationalities overtly in the beginning phase. Your client needs to learn about the existence of his overt irrational beliefs before he can deal with the covert ones.

How might irrational beliefs be expressed in your client's verbalisations? Early in therapy your client comes to a session one minute late and apologises profusely for his lateness. This may either indicate that he has an irrational belief concerning time or about possible rejection. Another client who is paying your fee and says at the end of a first session 'It was extremely good of you to see me' may be revealing a subtle irrational belief concerning approval. If you run group therapy sessions you may gain a lot of important information about the presence of subtle irrational beliefs by listening carefully to clients' exchanges with one another.

Implicit irrational beliefs may also be present in subtle forms of client behaviour. Take eye contact: some clients who hold shame-based irrational beliefs may reveal these beliefs when they adjust their eye contact at various point in the therapeutic or social dialogue. Of course, we all alter our eye contact during a conversation, but clients whose beliefs are shame-based may do so in order not to experience the disturbing emotion of shame; however, by doing so, they reveal and strengthen their irrational beliefs.

When your clients have made progress in changing their core irrational beliefs and have begun acting according to their new core rational beliefs, you may then draw their attention to the subtle operation of irrational beliefs in their everyday talk and behaviour.

> **Key point**
>
> *Be alert to the possible existence of hidden irrational beliefs in your clients' commonplace verbalisations and behaviours. Use such beliefs as part of your assessment early in therapy and consider dealing with them later in therapy after your clients have made progress in changing their more overt irrational beliefs.*

35 Allow for time-limited irrationalities in your clients

It is the case that a major goal of REBT is to encourage clients to make profound philosophical changes so that they can be as psychologically healthy as possible. However, only a very small minority of your clients will stay in therapy to achieve that level of psychological maturity. Most of your clients will be satisfied with more limited, and some would say, more realistic therapeutic objectives. If you are extremely ambitious for your clients in terms of what you think they can achieve, this may be at variance with what they actually seek from therapy. I believe that most people who do not have psychological problems or who do not seek therapeutic help for problems that they do have, experience what I call time-limited irrationalities. Thus, they may upset themselves for a time about an activating event, but after a short while they stand back and rethink the experience or focus on other aspects of their environment. They do not consider their time-limited disturbances a problem. Indeed, some individuals, and I would include myself here, may disturb themselves about an experience, but are able to put that experience in a more rational perspective.

I often tell my clients the following story. I was away from my house for the weekend and my neighbours rang up to tell me that there was a leak in my house since a large ice flow had appeared on the outside wall. My own reaction to this news was to make myself extremely upset at the prospect of my books being flooded out and ruined. For about 25 minutes I experienced a mixture of anger and anxiety, I ranted and raved, and kicked chairs around. Whether or not this experience was cathartic for me and whether or not I needed this experience in order to begin to think rationally are matters on which I cannot comment. What is important about this episode is that after a period of 25 minutes, I was able to think more clearly and more rationally. Note that I was in no frame of mind to use my REBT disputing skills on myself when I was so upset – a phenomenon clients frequently report on. Also, I was not ashamed of the fact that, even as an REBT therapist, I disturbed myself for a period of time. Rather I saw this reaction as being quite human and not necessarily unhealthy. Thus, I often explain to my clients that my job is not to help them eradicate all of their irrationalities, but only those they cannot quickly change. REBT is best used, therefore, when your clients get stuck with their irrational beliefs for an extended period of time and cannot do anything constructive about shifting them.

This principle particularly applies to grief. Many writers on grief have noted that clients experience a range of different emotions at different times when they lose a loved one. It may very well be that when your client is angry about her loss, she is thinking irrationally. It may also be that when she is searching for her loved one, she is thinking irrationally. However, my view is that if this reflects a time-limited irrationality, it is not necessarily helpful for you to intervene and help her to identify, challenge and change the irrational beliefs underlying her anger or searching behaviour. However, when your client becomes stuck in an extended grief reaction, either because she reminds herself frequently of her loss or because she studiously avoids going through a healthy grief and mourning process, then you can productively use REBT to help her deal with her unhealthy grief reaction.

> **Key point**
>
> *Do not become overly zealous in applying REBT to all of your clients' irrationalities. Allow them and yourself to have time-limited irrationalities.*

36 Guard against insensitivity when challenging your clients' irrational beliefs

If you use the rational emotive behavioural treatment sequence that Raymond DiGiuseppe and I published in 1990, when you have reached step 9 which involves disputing your client's irrational beliefs, then he ideally should have understood the relationship between these beliefs and his emotional and/or behavioural problem. When you dispute your client's irrational beliefs, use empirical, logical and pragmatic arguments to encourage him to surrender these beliefs and begin to help him to work towards constructing and deepening his conviction in an alternative set of rational beliefs. As you dispute your client's irrational beliefs, do so with sensitivity and tact since you are encouraging him to give up attitudes which, though self-defeating, are convincing to him. Help your client to understand that when you are disputing his irrational beliefs, you are attacking his beliefs and not him as a person. Encourage him to give you feedback on how he reacts to your disputing interventions.

There is a particular need for great tact and sensitivity when your client is disturbed about a traumatic event such as rape, sexual and other forms of abuse. In such circumstances, avoid using empirical arguments such as 'Where is the evidence that you absolutely should not have been raped or abused in this way?' Such arguments, by their very nature, may be construed as particularly insensitive and should, in my opinion, be avoided. Thus, when you dispute your client's irrational beliefs about abusive experiences, it is crucial that you show your client that you understand her emotional response and indicate that it is healthy to be very upset about such events. Your first task is to be empathic and your second task is to explain to her that you need to join together to help her give up her additional disturbance, but not her healthy upset. You need to convey repeatedly to the client that what she experienced *was* a catastrophe and even terrible which means, in this case, that she went through a very, very bad experience.

If you use the argument that such experiences were not awful and that worse things could happen, this will be experienced as, at best, an irrelevant argument and at worst an insensitive one, even though it is true according to REBT theory. This is particularly true when your client has been abused by a man and you are a male therapist.

> **Key point**
>
> *Use tact and sensitivity when disputing your clients' irrational beliefs, especially when they are disturbed about real-life tragedies.*

37 Assess the basis for client change

When your client reports improvement, it is important that you assess the basis for this change. Determine whether your client has improved by changing his irrational beliefs, by changing the distorted nature of his inferences, by avoiding certain problematic activating events, by changing his environment or by changing his behaviour without making corresponding changes in his thinking. In addition, look at the consistency of your client's improvement. Has he overcome his disturbed feelings together with showing improvement in his behaviour, or has one change occurred in the absence of the other?

When your client reports improved changes in his disturbed feelings and is now acting in a self-enhancing manner, if these changes are based on underlying attitude change, this is a most desirable outcome. However, if your client has effected changes by modifying aspects of his psychological functioning which do not involve belief change, then you need to reinforce those changes, but urge him to take that extra step and work at bringing about changes in his underlying irrational beliefs.

> **Key point**
>
> *When your clients report improvement, assess the bases for these changes. Encourage them to change their irrational beliefs if they have not already done so.*

38 Reinforce change without reinforcing your clients' need for approval

Following the lead of Albert Ellis, REBT therapists are, in general, quite careful not to reinforce their clients' need for approval. As such, we tend to avoid forming overly warm attachments with our clients or giving them lavish praise. However, in our zeal to avoid reinforcing our clients' need for approval, many of us fail to offer them sufficient encouragement to promote and maintain client change. Healthy encouragement for client change may take the form of you saying to your client: 'It was good that you achieved that', or 'I am pleased you were able to do that'. With some of your clients, you may wish to add a humorous and ironic statement such as: 'But that does not make you a better person', or 'But that does not mean I like you more'. If you give your client 'healthy encouragement', then you will serve as a useful role model for him, so that he can learn to encourage himself and praise his own actions as well as doing the same for others in his life.

When your client does not achieve much from his homework assignments, you still need to encourage him for making the effort. Here, it is important to distinguish between effort and the outcome of that effort. Thus, you might say to your client: 'I am sorry you were unable to achieve what we both hoped you might from the assignment, but I am encouraged by the fact that you really made the effort. Now, let's discover what obstacles, if any, there were which prevented you from achieving what we hoped you might.'

Even when your client fails to initiate change by consistently failing to do his homework assignments, you can still encourage him to do so by stressing his potential to change. You might say: 'The fact that you consistently refuse to do your homework assignments is a great shame, because you really could change if you worked at it.'

Let me conclude this point with a caveat. By all means encourage your client to change, but guard against encouraging your client to do what is beyond his potential to achieve.

> **Key point**
>
> *Guard against reinforcing your clients' need for approval when you reinforce their change-directed efforts. However, do not let this stop you from offering them healthy encouragement as they work (or struggle) towards rationality.*

39 Do not be afraid to be repetitive

Your clients will rarely, if ever, learn to surrender part of an irrational belief and gain deep conviction in a rational belief after one session. A client may understand a rational principle in one session and in the very next session act as if she has not even heard of that principle. It is important, therefore, to realise that you will need to repeat your interventions before your clients begin to understand and act on the rational principles that you teach them. With some clients, it is important to repeat rational messages in exactly the same way. For some reason, hearing the same rational message put the same way repeatedly is an important ingredient for those clients' understanding. With such clients, if you teach the same principle in different ways they will end up confused. So, ask your client whether he learns best by having the same material repeatedly presented in the same way or whether he finds it more useful to have the same thing taught in different ways. Your client's answer to this question is a useful pointer for the way you present rational principles, although it should not be regarded as an absolute indication.

Once you have established that your client learns best from variety, you should seek to repeat the same rational principle but using, for example, different explanations, a variety of analogies and audio-visual aids. Realise that with yet other clients you may need to keep varying the medium of your message until they indicate that a particular way of conveying the message is useful. In such a case, you will then need to repeat the rational principle using the client's favoured technique until he begins to act and internalise that principle.

> **Key point**
>
> *You will often need to repeat rational principles until your clients have learned to internalise them. Realise that some clients respond best to rational principles being taught in the same way, while other clients respond best to a more varied approach.*

40 When in doubt, return to first principles

Sheldon Kopp (1977) has written a very useful book called '*Back to one*'. He noted that as therapists become innovative practitioners they introduce a lot of variety and experimental interventions into their work. However, he makes the important point that some therapists may get carried away with their own creativity to the detriment of their work with clients. When this occurs, he suggests that therapists need to go 'back to one', by which he means returning to the fundamental principles which guide their work.

Although I value therapeutic creativity, I have occasionally been too innovative before a client has really grasped certain principles that are fundamental to the successful practice of REBT. Thus, I have sometimes omitted to formally teach a client the ABCs of REBT so that she fails to see clearly the effects of irrational beliefs on her emotional and behavioural problems. On other occasions, I have neglected to stress that I expect my clients to work actively to bring about change. When I have returned to first principles, therapeutic movement has occurred.

> **Key point**
>
> *Be creative in your practice of REBT, but do not neglect the fundamental principles of the therapeutic approach. If you get stuck or are in doubt as to how to proceed with your clients, go back to first principles, i.e. go back to one.*

41 Be flexible in terminating therapy

Your clients will terminate therapy in a number of ways. Sometimes they will do so in a planned manner, at other times termination will be unplanned. Given the variety of ways that therapy can end, you need to be flexible in the way that you plan terminating with your clients.

One way is to increase the interval between therapy sessions as a way of encouraging your clients to take increasing responsibility for their self-change process. Here, you exchange your role as therapist for that of consultant, where you encourage your client to use you when she is finding it difficult to apply her REBT skills to life's problems. This approach to termination may be a misnomer since therapy may not come to an end: your client may come back many years later for a one-off session or a brief number of therapy sessions. This model of termination is in accord with the work of Budman and Gurman (1988), who view therapy as an intervention to be used at different stages of a person's life cycle and particularly when clients experience difficulty in making the transition from one life stage to the next. In this model of termination, such sessions are best viewed as booster sessions in that they provide your clients with: (1) a short refresher course on rational principles that they may have overlooked or forgotten; (2) new ways of looking at these principles; or (3) further encouragement to keep using the skills that they had internalised earlier in the therapeutic process, but which may have become rusty.

A different approach to termination involves setting a specific ending date without correspondingly reducing the frequency of sessions (of course the two models of termination can be combined). Make use of this particular mode of termination when your clients are moving away from your geographical area or to another country. You may both realise that the client needs further therapeutic work, but that it is impractical for her to continue to see you. Under these circumstances you can suggest REBT therapists that your client may consult in her new location. The reason I do not myself often set specific dates for termination, is because it does not provide sufficient encouragement for clients to take responsibility for their self-change process and does not give them enough opportunity to become independent in their use of REBT skills.

There is also a type of termination which may be best called 'temporary termination'. Following this approach, you recognise that your client may not be ready to terminate therapy altogether, but that at present she is not facing any negative activating events. Consequently, she does not have much to work on in therapy. For example, a female client with a need for approval when she is in a relationship may cope perfectly well without a relationship and would require a new relationship to work productively on her approval issue. In order to work productively with this issue she needs the stimulus of a disturbance-triggering activating event. Thus, you may encourage her to terminate therapy temporarily and resume it as soon as she has begun a new relationship or when she finds herself in a situation which triggers her core irrational belief.

Finally, since ending a therapeutic alliance with your client is an important phase of therapy, be sure to discuss with him the best way to end the work you have done together.

> **Key point**
>
> *Be aware that there are different ways to terminate therapy with clients. Be flexible in terminating therapy with your clients and negotiate with each of them the best way to end.*

Part IV

Encouraging Clients to Work at Change

42 Let your clients' brains take the strain

Recently, there was an advertisement for British Rail which exclaimed 'Let the train take the strain'. This message was used to encourage travellers to leave their cars at home and to travel by train, the emphasis being that travelling by train could spare people the stress of travelling by car. Successful REBT depends, to a large degree, on the extent to which your client assumes active responsibility to help herself. Part of this responsibility involves the client thinking for herself and actively applying cognitive change techniques. Thus, REBT is a form of therapy that encourages clients to use their brains as well as acting on what they have learned.

However, since REBT is an active–directive approach to therapy, it is quite easy for you to do a lot of the work for your client, particularly when you didactically teach her rational principles. Whenever possible, then, try to work socratically with your client, and encourage her to think through issues for herself. However, if you do need to use didactic explanations, it is especially important to encourage your client to put into her own words her understanding of what you are trying to convey. This not only helps her to be actively involved in therapy, it also helps you to gain feedback on whether or not you are communicating clearly and whether or not your points are being thoughtfully internalised by your client.

One of the dangers of REBT that you need to guard against is that some clients who learn the principles of REBT do so parrot fashion. They hope that repeating the words to themselves will be sufficient to bring about change. However, as I say to my clients: 'I may be able to teach a parrot to sound rational but I am not able to teach a parrot to think rationally and independently for itself'.

Letting the client's brain take the strain or encouraging her to do the work is equally important once she has begun to use the REBT method of change in her own life. When this has begun to happen, rather than take an active–directive stance, use open-ended prompts to maximise the extent to which your client thinks things through for herself. For example, once your client has learned to use the ABCDEs of REBT, ask the following open-ended questions to stimulate her to apply this to her own problems:

'How did you feel on that occasion?'
'What was going through your mind at that time?'
'How did you dispute that?'
'What were the effects of that dispute?'

'How could you have disputed that in a different way?'
'Did you believe the outcome of your dispute?'
'Why not?'
'What might you believe instead?'
'How do you know that is true?'
'What could you do in order to strengthen that new belief?'
'How might you overcome that obstacle?'

Your client may not be able to answer these questions fully but at least when you ask her, you are encouraging her to think through for herself the issues concerned. You are letting her brain take the strain.

> **Key point**
>
> *Use every opportunity to encourage your clients to think through issues for themselves. Guard against your clients learning rational principles by rote. Let their brains take the strain.*

43 Help your clients to engage in relevant change-producing tasks

Both you and your client have your respective tasks to perform in REBT and the goals of therapy in part dictate the selection of the tasks your client needs to carry out in order to experience change. If you have a good bond with your client, this may make it more likely that the client will engage in these tasks. As well as keeping therapy goal-directed and developing and maintaining a good working relationship with your client, there are other points that you need to consider when encouraging your client to do his share of the work in therapy:

1. Ensure that the tasks which you are encouraging your client to carry out are understood by him and that he sees how engaging in these tasks can help him achieve his therapeutic goals.
2. Only suggest client tasks that have sufficient therapeutic potency, i.e. if the client performs them adequately, they have the power to lead to a good therapeutic outcome. Here, knowledge of the relevant research literature is important. For example, in the anxiety disorders, while the contribution of cognitive techniques to good outcome is still equivocal, exposure tasks do yield a good therapeutic outcome. Thus, if your client has an anxiety disorder, failure to use exposure techniques will make it less likely that your client will realise his goals.

3. Make sure that your client has the ability to engage in the relevant therapeutic tasks. Asking a client with limited IQ to complete a complex self-help form may end in failure, whereas asking a bright and sophisticated client to carry out an overly simple task may, from his perspective, insult his intelligence.
4. Consider the client's psychopathology when thinking of therapeutic tasks that he can carry out. As noted in Point 6 it may be counterproductive for you to ask your client to engage in a task which may otherwise have excellent therapeutic potency, if he considers it 'too overwhelming' for him at a given point in time. Thus, although a therapeutic task may be clearly indicated, it is perhaps more important to compromise with the client and encourage him to do what is feasible for him, rather than to press him to do something which he is unlikely to do.

In my experience, when REBT therapists press their clients too hard, their clients perceive them as insensitive and domineering, two qualities which are hardly conducive to a continuing productive working alliance. However, when a task is challenging for your client, but not overwhelming for him and he expresses concern about his ability to engage in that task, consider the three Cs. Your client may believe that, before he carries out the task, he first has to have sufficient *confidence*, experience sufficient *comfort* and he must be *certain* about what will happen. Disputing your client's demands for confidence, comfort and certainty is a pre-requisite to helping him engage in challenging, change- producing tasks.

> **Key point**
>
> *Consider a number of salient issues when thinking of suitable tasks that your clients can carry out to achieve their therapeutic goals.*

44 Use a variety of self-help forms

On a recent visit to the Institute for Rational-Emotive Therapy in New York, I was surprised to learn that training fellows there do not routinely encourage their clients to use a variety of self-help forms. It is my experience that such self-help forms serve several useful purposes in the therapeutic process:

1. They help your client to organise her experiences in a meaningful way. As such, they offer your client an opportunity to gain a sense of

control and counter her tendency to be overwhelmed by her experiences. This is particularly true if your client uses written self-help forms as soon as she begins to feel disturbed.
2. They remind your client that she is expected to help herself, that the effects of therapy do not come solely from attending therapy sessions and that there is much she can do to help herself between sessions.
3. They remind your client about the nature of her problems, the kind of factors that are relevant in maintaining these problems and what she can do in order to tackle them.

PROBLEMS AND GOALS RATING SCALES

Name:		Therapist:				
PROBLEMS — Choose a number between 0 and 10 to indicate how much you are upset about your problems, where 0 represents not at all upset and 10 represents extremely upset.			Date:			
A)			Rating:			
B)			Rating:			
C)			Rating:			
D)			Rating:			
GOALS — Choose a number between 0 and 10 to indicate your progress towards achieving your goal regularly without difficulty, where 0 represents 0% success and 10 represents 100% success.			Date:			
A)			Rating:			
B)			Rating:			
C)			Rating:			
D)			Rating:			

Figure 1 Problems and Goals rating scales.

Figures 1, 2 and 3 show three forms that I use regularly in my practice. The first is called 'Problems and Goals' (see Figure 1) and helps your client to specify succinctly what her problems are and what her goals are with respect to each problem. While helping your client to formulate her goals, encourage her to focus on those that are achievable, realistic and measurable. The section of the form which encourages your client to rate the intensity of her problems and to rate the progress she is making towards realising her goals should be completed periodically by the client (e.g. monthly) to enable her to monitor her rates of therapeutic improvement.

The written self-help form (Figure 2) was devised by Jane Walker, an ex-student, and myself and has two main features:

Encouraging clients to work at change 69

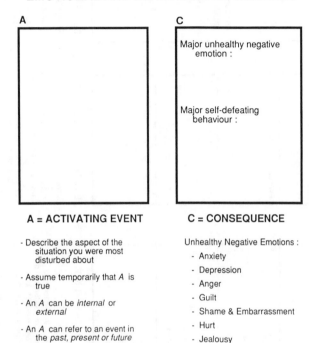

ABC
OF
EMOTIONAL AND BEHAVIOURAL PROBLEMS

A

C

Major unhealthy negative emotion :

Major self-defeating behaviour :

A = ACTIVATING EVENT

- Describe the aspect of the situation you were most disturbed about
- Assume temporarily that A is true
- An A can be *internal* or *external*
- An A can refer to an event in the *past, present or future*
- An A can be an *interpretation*

C = CONSEQUENCE

Unhealthy Negative Emotions :
- Anxiety
- Depression
- Anger
- Guilt
- Shame & Embarrassment
- Hurt
- Jealousy

Figure 2 ABC of emotional and behavioural problems (the A and C sections are completed first). (Copyright Windy Dryden and Jane Walker, 1992.)

1. The first page opens out to reveal the second page. This encourages your client to fill in the A and C before the iB section.
2. The form encourages the client to zero in on the four main irrational thinking processes and also helps her realise that there are also four main thinking processes which serve as rational alternatives to these irrational beliefs.
3. The form reminds your client of the three major arguments which she can use to dispute her irrational beliefs (i.e. empirical, logical and pragmatic arguments).

iBs

DOGMATIC DEMAND :
AWFULISING :
LOW FRUSTRATION TOLERANCE :
SELF/OTHER DOWNING :

iBs = IRRATIONAL BELIEFS

Look for :

- DOGMATIC DEMANDS (musts, absolute shoulds, oughts)
- AWFULISING (It's awful, terrible, horrible)
- LOW FRUSTRATION TOLERANCE (I can't stand it, I can't bear it)
- SELF/OTHER DOWNING (bad, worthless, less worthy)

D

Is it true? Is it logical? Is it helpful?
Is it true? Is it logical? Is it helpful?
Is it true? Is it logical? Is it helpful?
Is it true? Is it logical? Is it helpful?

D = DISPUTING

- Where is the evidence to support the existence of my irrational belief? Is it consistent with reality?
- Is my belief logical? Does it logically follow from my rational belief?
- Where is holding this belief getting me? Is it helpful?

rBs

NON-DOGMATIC PREFERENCE :
EVALUATING BADNESS :
HIGH FRUSTRATION TOLERANCE :
SELF/OTHER ACCEPTANCE :

rBs = RATIONAL BELIEFS

Strive for :

- NON-DOGMATIC PREFERENCES (wishes, wants, desires)
- EVALUATING BADNESS (It's bad, unfortunate)
- HIGH FRUSTRATION TOLERANCE (I can stand it, I can bear it)
- SELF/OTHER ACCEPTANCE ("Fallible human being" concept)

E

New healthy negative emotion :

New constructive behaviour :

E = NEW EFFECT

Healthy Negative Emotions :

- Concern
- Sadness
- Annoyance
- Remorse
- Disappointment
- Regret
- Concern about my relationship

Figure 2 (contd)

Task assignment form
Name: Date: Negotiated with:
AGREED TASK - State the task and when, where and how frequently you have agreed to do it:
THE THERAPEUTIC PURPOSE(S) OF THE TASK:
OBSTACLES TO CARRYING OUT THE TASK - What obstacles, if any, stand in your way of completing this task and how you can overcome them: 1. 2. 3. 4. 5.
WHAT I ACTUALLY DID AND LEARNED
Signed:

Figure 3 Task assignment form.

Figure 3 details the 'task assignment form', which encourages your client to make a written note of the homework assignment she has agreed to carry out between therapy sessions, the purpose of carrying out this assignment, what obstacles she might experience which may stop her from doing the assignment and what she can do to overcome these obstacles.

Finally, there is a section for her to detail what she has learned from carrying out the homework assignment.

Key point

Appreciate the value of self-help forms and use them to encourage clients to specify their problems and goals, dispute their irrational beliefs and carry out their homework assignments.

---

45 Systematically train your clients to use REBT self-help forms

Having made the case for the routine use of self-help forms in REBT, I want to stress that you need to train your client in their use. It is insufficient for you to give your client the form and tell him to fill it out. You need systematically to train him to use it. Consider using the following training steps, taking the ABC form presented in Figure 2 (see Point 44) as an example.

1. Work through a problem. This could usefully be from another client's experience. Help your client understand that A and C need to be completed before B, that there are four possible irrational beliefs to look out for in the iB section, that there are three questions to use when disputing these beliefs and that there are four rational beliefs to strive for under rB.
2. Repeat the modelling exercise with a worked example of one of your client's problems, preferably one that she has experienced recently, so that the relevant information is fresh in her mind.
3. Encourage the client to take another recent example of her problem and use the form for herself. Prompt the client as she goes through the form and briefly explain why she needs to place information in the suggested spaces.
4. Ask your client to complete the form on her own. If necessary, briefly leave your office to encourage her to do it for herself. This normally takes 10–15 minutes. When you return, read the completed form and give your client feedback on her responses, praise her effort and achievement and correct any errors she may have made.
5. Suggest that your client fills out two or three forms before the next therapy session as a homework assignment. Stress that as the form is quite difficult to master, you do not expect her to be competent at it for quite a while.

When your client has mastered the skills of completing the ABC form, show her that she can use it in one of two ways. She can do it as an intellectual exercise, by distancing herself from her emotions or she can get involved emotionally in the exercise. If she chooses the latter, she needs to get into the frame of reference of her new rational beliefs so she can experience the new healthy feelings that stem from such beliefs.

While there is, as far as I know, no experimental research that shows that training clients to fill in REBT self-help forms increases compliance, it is my experience that training does have this effect. Of course, as seasoned REBT therapists will appreciate, clients with a philosophy of low frustration tolerance may well fail to complete homework forms no matter how much preparation and training they are given!

> **Key point**
>
> *You can help your clients master self-help forms by systematically training them in their use. So, apply the five training steps that I have outlined in this section.*

46 Negotiate suitable homework assignments with your clients

Several studies suggest that clients who complete self-help homework assignments are more likely to improve than clients who do not (e.g. Burns and Nolen-Hoeksema, 1991). In addition, Burns and Nolen-Hoeksema (1992) found that clients who terminated therapy prematurely were less likely to complete self-help assignments between sessions than clients who remained in therapy. Thus the role of homework assignments in REBT and other approaches to cognitive behaviour therapy is not only theoretically important, but shown from empirical studies to be practically important in engaging clients in therapy and enhancing treatment gains. Consequently, pay particular attention to how you can encourage your client to complete homework assignments between sessions.

It is crucial that you negotiate suitable homework assignments with your client rather than unilaterally assign (or prescribe) them to her. I say this despite the fact that the superiority of a negotiating style to homework assignments as opposed to a unilaterally assigning style remains to be documented empirically. If you adopt such a negotiating style, then you need to bear in mind the following points:

1. Allocate sufficient time to negotiate assignments with your client, mainly at the end of therapy sessions.
2. A negotiating approach to homework tasks helps to avoid client reactance. When reactant clients are told to do something they often seek to regain their autonomy by resisting such authoritative influence. Consequently, asking such clients whether they could do something in between sessions to help themselves and discussing with them the potential usefulness of such tasks is preferable to telling them that they 'should' do something between sessions and that it *will* be helpful to them.
3. While negotiating a homework assignment with your client, help her see the relevance of undertaking such an assignment to achieving

her therapeutic goals. Also, you need to assess accurately her present capability to carry out the task. In addition, the more specific you can be with your client concerning which self-help assignment she needs to carry out, when she will carry it out, how frequently she will do it and in what context, the more likely it will be that your client will do the assignment.

4. Although you will most often negotiate a homework assignment with your client at the end of a session, it can also be the case that you will discuss such a task at the end of a piece of work in the middle of a session. When this is the case, it is still important that you review the agreed task at the end of the session. Have your client write the assignment down on a form such as the task assignment form (see Point 44, Figure 3) or on specially prepared homework prescription pads which have come into use as a result of work done on compliance in medical settings. This tends to show that when clients are given a written reminder of self-help steps, they are more likely to take these steps.

Over the course of REBT, different homework assignments will become more salient at different points in the therapeutic process. What follows is a discussion of a possible ordering of such assignments. This order is only illustrative and should not be regarded in any way as prescriptive. It is based on the most common sequence taken from a large number of therapy cases and may not apply to any given case.

At the beginning of REBT, encourage your client to carry out data-collection assignments (of thoughts, feelings, behaviours and troublesome activating events), particularly if she finds it difficult to identify such factors during therapy sessions.

Then, educational homework assignments may become particularly relevant. Suggest to your client that she reads books or excerpts from books or listens to tapes, to increase her comprehension of REBT principles. Tailor the suggested material to the comprehension level of the client and the client's particular problem. On this latter point, the books of Paul Hauck are particularly useful in that each is focused on a particular client problem, such as anger, depression and anxiety.

Next, you can introduce written self-help forms, particularly those which encourage your client to put her problems into the ABC framework (see Points 44 and 45).

Then you can employ imagery assignments to encourage your client to practise changing her feelings by changing her beliefs (as in rational-emotive imagery).

Finally, *in vivo* or behavioural assignments are particularly useful for helping your client deepen her conviction in her new rational beliefs by practising acting on them in real-life settings. If your client is prepared to carry out such behavioural assignments earlier in the process, then you could by-pass some of the prior steps discussed above.

As I discussed in Point 44, you need to pay particular attention to potential obstacles to the completion of a self-help assignment before your client attempts to carry it out. You need especially to assess the presence of low frustration tolerance beliefs as these frequently prevent your client from doing what she has agreed to do. However, there are numerous other obstacles to homework assignment completion and it is helpful to give your clients a checklist of such obstacles if non-compliance becomes an issue in therapy (see Appendix below, taken from Dryden, 1990a, for an example of such a checklist). This will help your client to identify her own obstacles to completing homework assignments.

> **Key point**
>
> *Since homework assignments play such a key role in facilitating client change, take great care to negotiate suitable assignments with your clients. Consider suggesting different assignments at different stages of the therapeutic process.*

Appendix: possible reasons for not completing self-help assignments

(To be completed by client)

The following is a list of reasons that various clients have given for not doing their self-help assignments during the course of counselling. Because the speed of improvement depends primarily on the amount of self-help assignments that you are willing to do, it is of great importance to pinpoint any reasons that you may have for not doing this work. It is improtant to look for these reasons at the time that you feel a reluctance to do your assignment or a desire to put off doing it. Hence, it is best to fill out this questionnaire at that time. If you have any difficulty filling out this form and returning it to the counsellor, it might be best to do it together during a counselling session. (Rate each statement by ringing 'T' (True) 'F' (False). 'T' indicates that you agree with it; 'F' means the statement does not apply this time.)

1. It seems that nothing can help me so there is no point in trying.   T/F
2. It wasn't clear, I didn't understand what I had to do.   T/F
3. I thought that the particular method the counsellor had suggested would not be helpful. I didn't really see the value of it.   T/F
4. It seemed too hard.   T/F

5. I am willing to do self-help assignments, but I keep forgetting.	T/F
6. I did not have enough time. I was too busy.	T/F
7. If I do something the counsellor suggests I do it's not as good as if I come up with my own ideas.	T/F
8. I don't really believe I can do anything to help myself.	T/F
9. I have the impression the counsellor is trying to boss me around or control me.	T/F
10. I worry about the counsellor's disapproval. I believe that what I do just won't be good enough for him/her.	T/F
11. I felt too bad, sad, nervous, upset (underline the appropriate word(s)) to do it	T/F
12. It would have upset me to do the homework.	T/F
13. It was too much to do.	T/F
14. It's too much like going back to school again.	T/F
15. It seemed to be mainly for the counsellors benefit.	T/F
16. Self-help assignments have no place in counselling.	T/F
17. Because of the progress I've made these assignments are likely to be of no further benefit to me.	T/F
18. Because these assignments have not been helpful in the past, I couldn't see the point of doing this one.	T/F
19. I don't agree with this particular approach to counselling.	T/F
20. OTHER REASONS (please write them).	

47 Encourage your clients to do daily self-help assignments

When people seek medical help from their general practitioners, they will frequently take their medication only until their condition improves, unless they have a chronic condition which necessitates taking on-going medication to prevent the return of symptoms. In therapy, when your client does homework assignments successfully, he may well stop carrying them out once his disturbed feelings and self-defeating behaviours diminish and he may not re-institute such assignments until he begins to experience his troublesome symptoms again.

To counteract this tendency, suggest to your client that he allocates a small period of each day to emotional self-help even though he may not be disturbed. The rationale I give for this is that continued self-help enables clients to internalise rational beliefs and consolidate the gains they have already achieved in therapy. Find out how much time your client spends on self-maintenance in the area of physical well-being (include time spent cleaning teeth, washing clothes and feeding etc.). Then ask your client what would happen if he did not carry out such maintaining behaviour. Your client will probably see, for example, that if he stops cleaning his teeth regularly, then his teeth and gums will deteriorate. Then ask him how much time he is prepared to allocate to the maintenance of his emotional well-being. If you can encourage your client to allocate, say, 15 minutes each day to self-help even though he is not disturbed, then this preventive work will be well worth the time investment.

Thus, encourage your client to complete an ABC form each day or to take a risk each day so that he can continue to practise consolidating his rational beliefs in challenging environments. This is particularly helpful for clients who have a philosophy of low frustration tolerance. If you can encourage them to commit themselves to a daily routine of emotional self-care, then they will not only get the benefit of carrying out such assignments, but they will also tend to raise their level of frustration tolerance.

> **Key point**
>
> *Encourage your clients to commit themselves to daily emotional self-care even if they do not feel disturbed.*

48 Regularly check homework assignments at the beginning of the next session

As I have shown in Point 47, your client needs to complete self-help assignments regularly if she is to benefit from REBT. To ensure that you convey the importance of homework, check on the assignments that your client carried out from the previous session. Do this normally at the beginning of the following session. Allocating sufficient time on the session agenda to check on homework assignments communicates to your client that you are taking their completion seriously.

If you encourage the use of the task assignment form (discussed in Point 44), have your client hand this to you at the beginning of each therapy session. This will help you to gauge quickly the outcome of your client's self-help endeavours. In particular, find out what your client learnt from the assignment and suggest ways in which she can consolidate such learning in the future.

If your client has agreed to do data-collection homework assignments, enquire what she has learnt from the data she has collected and also check to see if there are any gaps in the log that she kept. If there are such gaps, establish what difficulties the client experienced in collecting the material and suggest suitable remedies.

If you asked your client to carry out an educational homework assignment such as reading an excerpt from a book or listening to a tape, assess carefully what she learnt from the material. In particular, elicit any doubts or disagreements that the client had with the material. If your client does not disclose any doubts and disagreements that she may have, then she will continue to harbour them. However, if you bring them out into the open, then at least you have the opportunity to correct any misconceptions that the client may have about the material.

If your client agreed to complete one of the various written self-help forms that are available, then you need to go over it in a careful, step-by-step manner, correcting any errors that your client may have made in completing the form. Do so, however, within the broad context of reinforcing the client for what she has achieved and showing her encouragement for future use of the form.

If the client agreed to do an imagery assignment, then check whether she was able to imagine the negative activating event with sufficient vividness to enable her to gain practice at changing her irrational beliefs to rational beliefs. If she practises rational–emotive imagery, then you need to pay particular attention to whether she first made herself disturbed about the activating event before striving to change her disturbed feelings to more constructive negative feelings by spontaneously changing her irrational beliefs to rational beliefs. If not, encourage her to do this in a future assignment.

If the client carried out a behavioural assignment where the emphasis was on exposing herself to situations in which she practised identifying, challenging and changing her irrational beliefs, then a number of points become relevant. First, did she confront the activating event, get upset and then work towards overcoming her upset? If this was the case, did she achieve her emotional gains by challenging her irrational belief, modifying an inference or distracting herself from the most relevant part of the A? Did she use denial or did she overcome one upset by replacing it with another? For example, some clients manage to confront an anxiety-triggering activating event by becoming angry. If this was the case, help her to see how she can overcome her anxiety without making herself angry.

If your client did confront the troublesome activating event and did not get upset, then it is important to understand the reason for this. Was she able to refrain from disturbing herself by quickly challenging her irrational beliefs or was the activating event not a relevant one? If the latter, you may have made an assessment error which you need to correct.

Sometimes, your client will have agreed to carry out a behavioural assignment and confront a specific activating event, but claim later that the event did not occur that week. If this is the case, then you need to help your client understand that she can actively seek out the event and not wait passively for it to occur.

If your client carried out her homework assignment successfully and in fact achieved a good outcome by acting on a rational belief, then you need to reinforce her success strongly. Then you can help her see how she can practise the same belief in related settings. However, if she did not do her homework assignment, it is important that you assess the reasons for this, perhaps by using the ABC framework or by referring to the list of reasons for not completing homework assignments discussed in Point 46. If you discover that your client has not done a homework assignment for an already established reason, devote sufficient time to help her vigorously dispute the relevant irrational belief and then re-negotiate the assignment. If, however, you identify a new reason for her not completing the homework assignment, then devote sufficient time to help the client discover how she might overcome this obstacle before re-negotiating the same assignment.

If your client continues to fail to carry out self-help assignments, then consider using rewards and penalties. Following the lead of Ellis, you can encourage your client to forego a pleasurable activity until she has carried out the homework assignment and to penalise (rather than punish or denigrate) herself if she fails to carry it out. For particularly intransigent problems in this area, you may need to suggest drastic measures, although you should note that on both sides of the Atlantic it is illegal to burn money!

If your client is apprehensive about doing homework, introduce the idea of the no-lose homework assignment. Show her that if she does the homework assignment, that will be helpful because she will be working towards achieving her therapeutic goals. Then, show her that if she does not do her homework, this can also be productive because it reveals to her the extent to which she defeats herself and helps you both identify subtle and not so subtle irrationalities which may count for her failure to complete the assignments. In addition, discuss with your client the empirical research literature which shows that therapeutic outcome is correlated with the execution of self-help assignments and indicates that your client needs to take full responsibility for this area of self-change.

One helpful technique that I use to encourage resistant clients to do what they stubbornly refuse to do (in this case, their homework) is as follows. I ask them how they would deal with this issue if a loved one approaches them for help but refuses to take responsibility for helping himself. Once I have elicited from such clients the response that I am looking for, namely they would encourage their significant other to do the assignment even though they felt unconfident or for any other reason, I then point out to them that they can usefully follow their own advice. However, it should be pointed out that some clients will stubbornly refuse to do self-help assignments no matter what you might do and you need to accept this grim reality and not disturb yourself about it. This will help you to get on with the task of persisting with therapy under difficult circumstances.

> **Key point**
>
> *Convey the importance of homework assignments by regularly checking them at the following therapy session. Encourage your clients to build on their successes and learn from their failures in this central area of REBT.*

49 Build in generalisation

When your client is beginning to make progress at overcoming his irrational beliefs about specific problems, it may be tempting for you to assume that since he has understood how to identify, challenge and change his irrational beliefs in one context, he will naturally be able to do so in other contexts. While some of your clients will be able to do this spontaneously without your active help, most will need your help in generalising their learning from one situation to others.

Suppose, for example, that your client believes that she must gain the approval of her boss at work. In therapy, she has learned to identify, challenge and change this belief with the result that she experiences less dysphoric emotions and has become more assertive with her boss. Your next step is to encourage her to identify other people in her life whose approval she thinks she needs. Help her to specify and seek out situations that involve the possibility of incurring the disapproval of these significant others and help her to challenge her approval-related irrational belief in these situations using cognitive disputing methods and imagery methods. As you do this, reduce your level of activity and direction as the client demonstrates her increasing ability to generalise her learning (see Point 4). Then, help the client to identify other core irrational beliefs and encourage her to identify, challenge and change these, first in specific situations and then in a broader range of situations. As your client demonstrates an increasing ability to generalise her self-helping skills from one set of situations to others, you can then teach her general rules about the REBT approach to self-help. Thus, you can teach your client first to learn to identify self-defeating emotions and behaviours, then to search for the clinically relevant aspects of the activating event, thereby to identify the irrational beliefs that underpin her problems (these may be specific versions of more general core irrational beliefs). Then, your client can utilise her disputing skills and begin to strengthen her conviction in her new specific and core rational beliefs by using a variety of cognitive, emotive and behavioural techniques.

While you can teach some of your clients these general principles at an early stage in therapy and they will be able to apply them to a broad number of situations straightaway, most of your clients will need to learn specific REBT skills in specific situations before they are able to apply the general principles more broadly.

> **Key point**
>
> *Do not leave it to chance that your clients will generalise their learning from therapy. Build this into your broad therapeutic approach.*

Part V

Disputing

50 Assume that A is temporarily true

Using the REBT treatment sequence (Dryden and DiGiuseppe, 1990), you will assess the C and A elements of your client's problem before identifying his irrational beliefs. As I have already stressed (see Point 32), while assessing A, you need to determine the most clinically relevant aspect of the activating event (i.e. that part of A that triggers the client's irrational belief). Once you have done this, you need to encourage your client to assume temporarily that A is true, no matter how distorted A is. The one major exception to this rule occurs when you think that your client is quite unlikely to think rationally about a very distorted A (e.g. when a client with panic disorder infers that she is going to die). In this case, you need to educate your client concerning the effect of the role that irrational beliefs have in producing distorted inferences and select an irrational belief lower down the client's chain of disturbance (see Point 21 for a fuller discussion of this issue).

Leaving this exception aside, encourage your client to assume temporarily that A is true. Why? Because it enables you to identify the irrational belief that triggered the client's emotional or behavioural problem. At this stage, if you encourage your client to challenge his inferential distortion you may indeed help him, but you will not get at the underlying irrational belief. Novice REBT therapists, in particular, find it difficult to resist disputing inferential distortions, particularly when these are clearly exaggerated. They may even believe that these distorted As really did cause the client's problem at C. This temporary amnesia for the ABC model of REBT can be frequently (but not always) explained by the novice therapist believing that she would be disturbed if she was confronted by this distorted A.

Let me illustrate some of these points by taking the example of Lisa, a jealous client. She says to you 'I'm sure that my husband is having an affair because I have discovered purchases on his credit card which I cannot account for'. It is very tempting at this point for you to dispute her A and ask such questions as 'What other reasons might there be for the unexplained purchases on his credit card?'. 'If he discovered some unexplained purchases on your credit card would that automatically mean that you were having an affair?'. While you will not wish to neglect disputing the A, do this after you have disputed the client's irrational beliefs. This strategy is recommended on the theoretical principle that irrational beliefs, when dogmatically held, encourage clients to make distorted interpretations of their environment. If you first help Lisa to see that her inferences about the situation are distorted and encourage her to be more realistic in her interpretations, then you have missed the opportunity of identifying and challenging the underlying irrational beliefs which really are at the core of her jealousy.

Realise also that Lisa will be more likely to challenge her distorted interpretations if she is in a more objective frame of mind to do so. You can best encourage her to achieve this frame of mind by helping her to become relatively undisturbed about her A through challenging her irrational beliefs.

> **Key point**
>
> *Encourage your clients, whenever practicable, to assume that their distorted inferences are temporarily true as a way of identifying and thence disputing their irrational beliefs.*

51 Dispute one irrational belief at a time

REBT theory states that when your client holds an irrational belief, this may have four major variants. First, and as Albert Ellis argues, primarily, the client holds a demanding 'must' about the A. Then, he may have one or more of three major derivatives from this 'must'. He may hold: (1) an awfulising belief; (2) a low frustration tolerance belief (e.g. 'I can't stand it'); and (3) a condemnatory belief applied to self, others or the world. Once you have determined that your client has one or more of these irrational beliefs, you are in a position to help him dispute them.

As you do so, help your client to dispute one irrational belief at a time. Thus, if your client understands that he does hold a 'must' about an activating event and can see the relationship between this 'must' and his disturbed emotion, help him to dispute this irrational belief until he can understand that the belief *is* irrational and that there is a rational alternative to it. This process requires the client's full attention and therefore you need to minimise anything that interferes with his full attention. If you switch from disputing your client's 'must', to disputing one of the other irrational belief variants before you have helped the client to dispute the 'must' fully, you will very likely confuse the client. The consequence of this confusion is that the client will neither adequately challenge his 'must' nor its derivative.

Novice therapists, in particular, make the mistake of switching among the four irrational beliefs in the conviction that disputing is a relatively brief intervention in which clients can be helped very quickly to understand the irrationality of their irrational beliefs and the rationality of their new rational beliefs, and can easily apply this learning. If this mistake is made, the client is effectively being asked to answer four questions at the same time – a situation which is quite conducive not only to client confusion, but also to client termination!

Another situation in which you may be tempted to switch from one irrational belief to another is when you have identified ego-related irrational beliefs and discomfort-related irrational beliefs. Guard against the temptation of switching from ego iB's to discomfort iB's and back again, since this will also lead to client confusion.

What I advocate is that you dispute one irrational belief at a time and do not switch until your client has gained full understanding of the irrationality of the irrational belief and the rationality of the alternative rational belief. There is only one major exception to this rule. Some clients find it easier to dispute, say, an awfulising belief than a demanding belief. If you have really encouraged your client to dispute a 'must' and she has not made any progress on this, then it may be productive to switch from the demanding belief to the awfulising belief. In some circumstances, once you have helped your client to challenge and change her awfulising belief, she may be more open to disputing her demanding belief.

> **Key point**
>
> *Dispute one irrational belief at a time. Avoid, whenever you can, switching your disputes among different irrational beliefs and creating client (and therapist!) confusion.*

52 Keep your clients' goals in mind while disputing

As discussed in Part I of this book, the effective practice of REBT is done within the context of a developing productive therapeutic alliance. One of the major components of the alliance is the client's goals for change (see Point 9). One of the most powerful motivators for encouraging your client to change her irrational belief is the extent to which her new rational belief helps her to achieve her goal. Salesmen have known for many years that potential customers will not buy a product that they think will not help them realise an important goal. I believe this is the same with psychotherapy. Therefore, keep your client's goal for change clearly at the front of her mind while disputing. Although logical and empirical disputes are valuable in the disputing process (as will be shown in the next point), helping your client to assess the pragmatic value of her presently held irrational belief as compared to the value of the alternative rational belief is often the key to the success of a disputing intervention.

You can determine the power of pragmatic disputes by only using logical and empirical disputes during a disputing sequence. Then add pragmatic disputes at the end of this sequence by bringing the client's goal into the discussion to see what difference pragmatic disputing makes. Given that human beings are goal-directed organisms, I think you will find that the disputing process is more personally meaningful for clients when goals are introduced. Although human beings are somewhat concerned with thinking that is logical and consistent with reality, they are far more interested in achieving their personally held goals. I am not suggesting that you neglect the use of logical and empirical disputes. What I am *strongly* advocating is that you particularly use pragmatic disputes and that you keep your client's attention fixed on how her irrational beliefs impede her from achieving her goals and how alternative rational beliefs may encourage her to achieve those goals.

> **Key point**
>
> *While disputing your clients' beliefs, stress how thinking rationally will encourage them to achieve their goals.*

53 Be comprehensive in disputing

When challenging your client's irrational beliefs, you can use logical, empirical and pragmatic disputes, each targeted at the four irrational belief processes (i.e. demandingness, awfulising, low frustration tolerance, and self/other downing).

Raymond DiGiuseppe (1991), in a seminal article on disputing, has argued that REBT therapists need to be comprehensive in their disputing interventions. In addition to outlining the irrational belief processes and types of arguments used (as described above), he has outlined four disputing styles and two major levels of abstraction at which irrational beliefs can be disputed.

With respect to disputing styles, REBT advocates a socratic style where you ask your client questions and encourage her to consider issues concerning whether and why a belief is rational or irrational. The way the client responds to your question then forms the basis for further open-ended questions and this dialogue persists until your client understands why her irrational beliefs are irrational and why her rational beliefs are rational. However, some clients may not respond well to socratic disputing, or at other junctures in the disputing process you may need to impart information in a different way if the socratic dialogue is to be resumed. Under these conditions, you should employ didactic disputing. This involves giving explanations about why irrational beliefs are indeed irrational and why rational beliefs are rational. You not only need to ensure that you convey accurate information, but also that your client understands the information that you give to her. So when you provide the client with didactic explanations, ask her to put into her own words her understanding of what you are conveying to her.

DiGiuseppe (1991) mentions two additional disputing styles: metaphorical and humorous. In metaphorical disputing, you tell your client a story, metaphor or analogy which conveys information concerning the rationality of a given belief that is embedded in the story etc. For example, Albert Ellis often tells his clients the story of two Buddhist monks who, while making a journey, come to a stream. There they meet a young woman who asks to be carried over the stream. The younger monk is first surprised and then disturbed that the older monk offers to pick her up to carry her across the stream, since their faith forbids physical contact with members of the opposite sex. After they have said goodbye to the woman and many hours later, the young monk plucks up the courage to ask his older master the reason for his forbidden behaviour. 'Master' he said, 'how is it that you held this woman, her breasts against yours, her bare arms against yours, and carried her across the stream when we are forbidden to do so?'. The old monk replied laconically 'My son, you're still carrying her'.

The point of this story is, of course, that as long as a client makes a demand that she must not do something which is forbidden, then she is preoccupied in an anxious and disturbed way with her behaviour. But, if she recognises that she can follow useful guidelines in a non-absolutistic, flexible way, then she can act against these guidelines if it is for a greater good.

When you dispute your client's irrational beliefs metaphorically, it is crucial that you check your client's understanding of your message. Thus, if your client had said, in response to your enquiry concerning what he gained from the story, that one must never carry women across streams, then the rational point of the story would have been lost. The advantage of metaphorical disputes is that they are memorable and if the client makes the right connection between the story and the appropriate rational principle, then they can have quite a lasting impact. However, if this connection is not made or remembered, then these disputes have limited utility.

The final style mentioned by DiGiuseppe (1991) is one that is humorous. Humorous disputes are frequently paradoxical in nature, in that you take your client's ideas to some ridiculous extreme without ridiculing him. The obvious purposes of humorous disputes are to encourage your client not to take himself and his ideas *too* seriously, and to gain a healthy distance from his irrationalities. Ellis' famous (or infamous) rational humorous songs are excellent examples of this type of dispute in style in that they are humorous, paradoxical, memorable, if not tuneful (Dryden, 1990b).

I have added a fifth disputing style to the four described by DiGiuseppe and which I call enactive disputing. Here, you demonstrate a rational principle by action. For example, if I am trying to dispute an irrational self-downing belief with a client, I may suddenly take a half glass of water and throw it over myself and ask my shocked client whether that was a stupid thing to do. If he says 'Yes', I follow this up with 'Does that make me a stupid person?'. As this example shows, enactive disputes can be dramatic, eye-catching and engaging. However, you need to ensure once again that the rational principle is remembered and therefore you need to ask your client about the point she thinks you have made. Otherwise, she will remember your dramatic action and forget the rational principle that you intended to demonstrate.

Needless to say, it is important that you think carefully about the style of disputing you are going to use with your clients and elicit feedback from them concerning the impact that these different styles have on them.

The final component in a comprehensive approach to disputing discussed by DiGiuseppe concerns the level of abstraction at which disputing is conducted. Irrational beliefs can vary from the very specific (e.g. 'I must be loved by Susan, my girlfriend, when I have shown her that I care for her'), to the very abstract (e.g. 'I must be loved by all significant people in my life at all times'). Most of the time you will start off disputing your client's specific irrational beliefs before moving to her more core general beliefs (although as shown in Point 33, this is not universally true). The important thing to remember here is that irrational beliefs occur at different levels of abstraction and you need to dispute both specific and general iB's at different times in the therapeutic process.

Key point

DiGiuseppe's scheme for the comprehensive disputing of irrational beliefs shows that the process of disputing can be quite complex. However, it provides you with flexibility concerning the type of arguments you can use in disputing, the style in which disputing can be carried out, the different irrational belief targets that you can aim at during disputing and the varying levels of abstraction at which you can work. If you are a novice REBT therapist, do not yet expect to be competent in all of these areas. As you gain in experience and as you learn from supervision, you will become more proficient in all the areas of disputing discussed in this point.

54 Be meaningful, vigorous and persistent in disputing

Michael Edelstein, an REBT therapist working presently in San Francisco, advocates the principle of 'MVP' in disputing: M stands for Meaningful, V for Vigorous and P for Persistent.

Making your disputing strategies meaningful for your client is important if you are to engage him fully in the disputing process. Thus, if you choose your metaphors, anecdotes, and analogies carefully to fit your client's life situation, interests, hobbies etc., then your disputes are likely to have greater meaning for him than if you use them without due regard for the client's likely response.

A good example of meaningful disputing is found in the work of Howard Young (Dryden, 1989b). Young was working with a man who had become disabled and could only work part-time, and who was putting himself down for his disability and for working less than full-time. Having established that the client was interested in baseball, Young proceeded in a way that shows clearly how he made his dispute meaningful for the client.

Young: Who's your favourite baseball player?
Client: Pete Rose! He's number one!
Young: Why?
Client: He's Charlie Hustle, He gives it all and never quits. You can depend on him when the chips are down.
Young: Let me ask you something – suppose Pete Rose, while sliding into third base, hurt his back so bad he could never play full-time again. He stays in baseball, but only as a pinch hitter. He never plays complete game innings. Would you think less of him and consider him a weakling?
Client: No! He'd be doing what you'd expect: playing until they rip his uniform off.
Young: But not full-time – he'd be a part-time player, right?
Client: Yeah.
Young: And you'd still respect him as a man even though he was part-time?
Client: Yeah, he'd still be valuable and important to his team but in a different way.
Young: So why can't you see yourself in the same way? You were once a full-time worker, but now, because of an injury, you gotta pinch hit – you're still pretty valuable, or the company wouldn't want you around – so why consider yourself a weakling?

Client: Yeah, I see what you mean – that's a good way to look at it. I'm still in the game, only now it's as a pinch hitter. I never thought of it in that way, comparing myself to Pete Rose and baseball. When you put it that way, it seems kind of silly to get down on myself.

The importance of being vigorous in disputing your client's irrational beliefs has been shown by Ellis, who has argued that you often need to be forceful, energetic and vigorous in your disputing if it is to be effective (Dryden, 1990b). What Ellis means by vigour in this context needs to be understood in the context of the strong and vigorous way that clients often cling to their irrational beliefs. Disputing your client's vigorously held irrational beliefs in a soft, gentle and weak manner is unlikely, Ellis claims, to help the client surrender these beliefs. Rather, you need to fight fire with fire and counter the vigour in which your client adheres to his irrational beliefs with a vigorous disputing manner. Of course, when you vigorously attack your client's irrational beliefs you need to make it clear that you are not vigorously attacking your client. Explain this to your client and get feedback from him concerning his reaction to your vigorous disputing strategies. Finally, when you use a vigorous style of disputing, you serve as a good role model for your client to use a vigorous style of self-disputing of his irrational beliefs.

Finally, it is important for you to be persistent when you dispute your client's irrational beliefs. As discussed in Point 39, you need to be repetitive when teaching your client rational principles. Applying this to the disputing process, you need to realise that your client is unlikely to surrender his irrational beliefs as a result of a single disputing episode, no matter how meaningful and vigorous that dispute may be. Rather, you need to repeat your disputing strategies many times either in the same way or in different ways.

Key point

When disputing your clients' irrational beliefs, do so persistently, with vigour and in a way that is most meaningful for them.

55 Use time-tripping imagery as part of your disputing strategy

When you dispute your clients' irrational beliefs, you will find that some rigidly cling to those beliefs, especially when the relevant A has just happened or might happen in the near future. When this happens, use time-tripping imagery (Lazarus, 1984) as a way of showing your client that what she may be presently disturbed about may in time be viewed differently and more rationally.

Let me provide an example to underscore this point. One of my clients was very anxious about being rejected by her boyfriend and was convinced that if she was rejected by him, then she would fall apart and would never recover. I asked her to imagine that she was in fact rejected by her boyfriend and that she was in fact extremely distraught about this. I then suggested that she imagine herself entering a time machine which could quickly take her into the future. I first asked her to imagine how she would feel a week after the rejection. She replied that she would still be distraught, depressed and suicidal. I then asked her to advance time one month into the future. She thought that she would be depressed and that life would still not be worth living. However, when she saw herself six months into the future, she began to see that she could put the event into a broader prospective, that life was not so bad after all and that she could begin to see a future for herself and even consider the possibility of dating another man. Having established that she could think rationally about this rejection, the issue was now: how long was it productive for her to think irrationally about it? What could she do to think more rationally about it sooner? She thought about this and concluded that perhaps she could be more rational about it three weeks after the rejection. I thought, in the circumstances, that this was reasonable and allowed her to have a time-limited irrationality (see Point 35).

> **Key point**
>
> *When your clients rigidly hold on to their irrational beliefs about an event that has just happened (or might happen) and do not respond to standard disputing techniques, add time-tripping imagery to the disputing process and help them see that they can think rationally about the event if it is progressed far enough into the future. Having made the point, show them that they can think rationally about it sooner rather than later.*

56 Discover and use disputing techniques that work for you

As you gain greater experience in REBT and get supervised in your work by different REBT supervisors, you will discover disputing techniques that are particularly successful with a wide variety of clients. Here I present two such disputing techniques which I have personally found quite useful in conveying important rational principles to clients.

The 'friend dispute'

Purpose: To dispute self-downing

The purpose of the 'friend dispute' is to help the client to see that she has a more tolerant and compassionate attitude towards a good friend than she has toward herself. From here the therapist can encourage the client to adopt this same tolerant and compassionate attitude toward herself. It is the rational emotive behavioural version of 'how to be your own best friend' and is best employed with self-downing issues. An example follows:

> Therapist: So can you see that you are saying to yourself that because you've lost your job you are a failure and that this leads to your depression?
> Client: Yes.
> Therapist: Now I'm going to help you re-evaluate that belief. What' the name of your best friend?
> Client: Mary.
> Therapist: Now let's suppose that Mary came to you and told you that she had lost a job that she valued. Would you say to her 'Get out of my house – you're a failure'?
> Client: No, of course not.
> Therapist: Would you think of her as a failure?
> [This is an important step to include in case the client would *think* of her friend as a failure even though wouldn't actually *say* this.]
> Client: No.
> Therapist: How would you think of her in the event of her losing her job?
> Client: Well, it wouldn't change my view of her. Even if she made a bad error she'd still be the same Mary.
> Therapist: The same fallible Mary?
> Client: Of course.
> Therapist: So let me get this straight. Mary loses her job and she's the

same fallible Mary. You lose your job and you are a failure.
Client: I see what you're saying.
Therapist: Now how about being consistent? Either you begin to view yourself as fallible or you start viewing Mary and other people as failures if they fail.
Client: So you are encouraging me to accept myself as fallible, as I would other people?
Therapist: That's right. Up to now, you have, in effect, been saying Mary is allowed to fail but *I'm* not. But if you give up the demand that you must not fail then you will begin to treat yourself as your own best friend.

The terrorist dispute

Purpose: To dispute awfulising and low frustration tolerance beliefs

The purpose of the 'terrorist dispute' is to help a client understand that he can stand or tolerate conditions or situations he thinks are unbearable and that many situations often are worth tolerating. An example follows:

Therapist: Okay, so we're clear now that what's frightening about going to the party is the prospect of spilling your drink and drawing people's critical attention to you.
Client: If that happened it would be unbearable. I'm getting anxious now, even thinking about it.
Therapist: So in your mind it would be terrible.
Client: Right on the button.
Therapist: Well, let's see if you're right. Do you love your children?
Client: Of course I do. What kind of question is that?
Therapist: Well, bear with me for a moment since I want to help you really think about whether or not your explanation of that scene we've just identified as 'terrible' is correct. Okay?
Client: Okay.
Therapist: Right. Now let's imagine that a group of terrorists capture your children and their ransom demand is this: 'If X (name of client) goes to 20 parties, spills a drink at each one, and thereby attracts the critical attention of others, we'll release his children. But if he doesn't do this we'll keep them forever.' Now would you do as they say?
Client: Of course I would.
Therapist: But you've just told me that even if you spill a drink once and are disapproved of once, then that would be terrible. How can you do something that is terrible?
Client: I'm beginning to see what you mean.

Therapist: What would you tell yourself about doing it 20 times to enable you to do it?
Client: That it's not *that* bad.
Therapist: That's right, that it is tolerable and presumably that it's worth tolerating in order to save your kids.
Client: Right.
Therapist: Now if you would do it 20 times to save your kids, will you risk it happening a couple of times for your mental health?
Client: Yes.
Therapist: And don't forget to practise convincing yourself that if the worst happens and you do spill a drink and attract criticism from others, then that is **bearable** and not terrible.

Key point

Discover disputing techniques that work for you. Experiment with other people's techniques (e.g. the 'best friend' and 'terrorist' disputes) and invent and test your own.

---

57 Help your clients to not only weaken their irrational beliefs but also construct and strengthen rational alternatives

Many novice REBT therapists think that the purpose of disputing is to help their clients realise that there is no evidence in support of their irrational beliefs. While this is one of the objectives of disputing, it is by no means the only one. There are several other additional tasks to be completed.

Having helped your client understand that there is no evidence in support of his irrational belief, you need to help him to construct a plausible rational alternative. This should preferably be expressed in the client's own words and he needs to see that holding this belief will help him to achieve his therapeutic goals (see Point 52). Having helped your client to construct a rational belief, your next task is to help him to weaken his conviction in his irrational belief and strengthen his conviction in the rational alternative.

Cognitively, you need to encourage your client not only to dispute his irrational belief but also to affirm his conviction in his rational belief. Behaviourally, you need to encourage your client to act according to his newly constructed rational belief while simultaneously negating his conviction in his irrational belief. Emotively, you need to encourage the client to use cognitive and behavioural strategies in a vigorous, passionate way so that his feelings are fully engaged. The more the client works to uproot his irrational belief and practise his new rational belief using cognitive, emotive and behavioural techniques, the more he will integrate his rational belief into his everyday emotional problem-solving repertoire.

Finally, the more the client challenges each of the four irrational belief variants (discussed in Point 51) and affirms each of the four rational alternatives, the more comprehensive his change in philosophy will be.

> **Key point**
>
> *For clients to change their philosophy, they need to both weaken their irrational beliefs and construct and strengthen their rational beliefs. The more they use cognitive, emotive and behavioural techniques, the greater the likelihood that their rational beliefs will make a difference in their lives.*

58 Encourage your clients to use a coping model of disputing rather than a mastery model

It will frequently be difficult for your clients to use the skills of disputing irrational beliefs and you therefore need to encourage them to be realistic in what they can expect from disputing. In my experience, clients, especially those with perfectionistic tendencies, expect that they will be able to master the skills of disputing quite quickly and use them without difficulty. They expect, for example, to be able to dispute irrational beliefs easily even though they are very upset, and further expect to feel comfortable in disputing their irrational beliefs.

In reality, there are several difficulties that virtually all of your clients will encounter when they start disputing their irrational beliefs. First, and particularly when your client is beginning to learn disputing skills, she will find it extremely difficult to dispute her irrational beliefs while she is feeling upset and disturbed. Here, you might urge her to reduce the level of her disturbed feelings by briefly distracting herself from them or by engaging in various self-soothing activities, before returning to disputing. Once your client has begun to internalise the skills of disputing, she will be better able to use disputing skills in the midst of an intense, emotional, upsetting experience. However, even then, particularly when she is feeling intensely anxious, she may not be able to do it. Prepare her for this eventuality and show her that she may need to reduce the intensity of her anxiety by staying with it and not fighting it. When the intensity drops, she may then return to disputing.

Many of your clients will report that when they try to dispute their irrational beliefs, they often do not 'feel right' or comfortable doing so or that they do not believe their new rational beliefs. They are strongly tempted to abandon disputing as a result. Maxie Maultsby (1984) has called this phenomenon 'cognitive–emotive dissonance' and explains the awkwardness that clients will inevitably experience when trying to believe a rational belief when at the same time they really believe the opposing irrational belief. Encourage your client to persist with disputing even though she is feeling awkward and even though she may not believe her new rational belief. Stress that this is an almost universal experience in the REBT change process. To borrow the intriguing title of Susan Jeffers' book *Feel the Fear and Do It Anyway* (Jeffers, 1987), I encourage my client to 'feel the awkwardness and dispute the belief anyway'.

When your client is beginning to learn to dispute her irrational beliefs, it is helpful to outline for her a sequence that she can realistically expect to go through and which represents a coping model of disputing as opposed to a mastery model. Have her notice when she is beginning to become emotionally upset and suggest that she use this as a cue to identify her irrational beliefs. Next, encourage her to struggle to dispute these beliefs and to work towards constructing a new rational belief. As she does so, urge her to feel the more healthy negative feeling that stems from this new rational belief. The coping model of disputing emphasises that your client needs to persist with disputing even though it is a struggle, and that it is worthwhile persisting if she is to derive emotional benefits. This model contrasts with the mastery model of disputing, where persistence and struggle are absent and where your client easily believes her new rational belief and thereby gains emotional benefit quickly and easily.

> **Key point**
>
> *Help your clients understand that they need to persist at disputing their irrational beliefs and that doing so is a struggle and often involves tolerating uncomfortable feelings. Contrast this coping model of disputing with a mastery model that, in reality, does not exist.*

59 Encourage your clients to identify and dispute for themselves the irrational beliefs of others

It is often helpful to encourage your client to use REBT with others. This involves your client engaging other people in a dialogue where she puts forward a rational belief and other people put forward an opposing strongly held irrational belief. The purpose of this technique is to give your client the practice of defending her rational belief against the attacking arguments of those who are defending their own related irrational beliefs.

A similar technique, and one that is less frequently used, involves encouraging your client to identify silently and dispute for herself the irrational beliefs that she hears either overtly or covertly expressed by others. Initially, you may encourage your client to do this by listening to radio and watching TV programmes, especially soap operas, where irrationalities are quite freely expressed. Have your client write down and dispute for herself the irrationalities that she hears and encourage her to develop new rational beliefs as healthy alternatives. You can also suggest that your client listens to the words of popular songs with the purpose of identifying irrational beliefs in the lyrics and rewriting the words of these songs to express rational beliefs. Thus, your client could change the words of the song 'You're No One until Someone Loves You' to 'You're Someone even though Nobody Loves You'. This assignment is not only instructive, but your client will probably find it entertaining.

After your client has had the opportunity of disputing irrational beliefs as expressed by characters on radio or TV, or as articulated in the lyrics of popular songs, encourage her to spend some time listening to her friends and relatives, noting and silently disputing the irrational beliefs articulated by these people. At this point, do not suggest that your client engage these significant others in a discussion about their irrationalities. When your client has gained experience of identifying and disputing the irrationalities of present and past significant others, this will help her to see that other people also have irrational beliefs and this will encourage her to be more sceptical of the source of those irrationalities rather than to assume that the source was correct. If, for example, your client reports that she has never been able to live up to the expectations of her father, encourage her to speculate about which irrational beliefs her father held and have her dispute them. This provides the impetus for your client to dispute her own irrational beliefs since she can now see that her father was in error concerning his expectations of her. As one of my clients reported, 'For the first time I can see that my father believed that I had to do well at school to make up for his own inadequacies as a father'. She proceeded to dispute her own irrational beliefs and concluded that she did not wish to make up for his inadequacies. Further, she came to believe that she and her father were both fallible human beings and that if her father was disappointed in her, this was more a reflection of her father's irrational beliefs than it was of her performance at school. Helping clients to dispute the irrationalities of significant others, particularly those that had a great influence on them in the past, is still a neglected area in REBT, even though I wrote my first REBT paper on this subject in the late 1970s (Dryden, 1979).

> **Key point**
>
> *One useful way of encouraging your clients to dispute their irrational beliefs is to have them identify and dispute those beliefs as they are expressed by others.*

60 Avoid premature and delayed disputing

While you do not have to use disputing strategies at just the right time in the therapeutic process, you do need to accomplish certain tasks before using these strategies. As Ray DiGiuseppe and I showed when we devised the rational emotive behavioural treatment sequence (Dryden and DiGiuseppe, 1990), before you can effectively dispute your client's irrational beliefs, you need to: (1) identify your client's target problem; (2) assess a specific example of that problem using the ABCs of REBT; (3) help your client to see the relationship between his irrational beliefs and his disturbed emotions and self-defeating behaviour at C; and (4) elicit your client's understanding that he can best achieve his therapeutic goals by disputing his irrational beliefs. Frequently, I have heard novice REBT therapists dispute their clients' irrational beliefs as soon as they hear these articulated by their clients. They have done so before they have properly prepared their clients to benefit from disputing. This premature or 'knee jerk' type of disputing very frequently leads to understandable client resistance and needs to be avoided whenever possible.

A different problem occurs when novice REBT therapists hold back on using disputing techniques. Rather than disputing their clients' irrational beliefs prematurely, these therapists delay their disputing interventions sometimes indefinitely. Instead of disputing irrational beliefs, these novice therapists: (1) encourage their clients to provide more information about them; (2) explore detailed nuances of their clients' feelings at C; or (3) engage their clients in an exploration of similar ABCs that are related to their target problems. In my experience, such REBT therapists are either fearful of making a mistake in the disputing process and therefore stay with what they are comfortable doing, or have previously been trained in forms of therapy that discourage therapists from challenging their clients. Therapists in the first category need to overcome their fear of failure by identifying and challenging their own fear-related irrational beliefs and using disputing strategies even if they do so poorly. They also need to understand that disputing is a high-level skill that can only be acquired through use with clients and through expert supervision. Therapists in the latter category need to ask themselves what they think will happen if they challenge their clients' irrational beliefs, and then test out their predictions by disputing these beliefs and eliciting their clients' reactions to their disputing interventions.

> **Key point**
>
> *Do not use disputing interventions until you have prepared your clients for their use. Having prepared your clients, do not delay using these interventions.*

61 Carefully distinguish between disputing questions and assessment questions

Whenever you are disputing your client's irrational beliefs, distinguish between questions designed to encourage the client to rethink these beliefs and questions designed to help you assess more carefully the inferential part of the A.

For example, consider a client who has the following irrational belief, 'My girlfriend must not pry into my affairs'. If you were to use a disputing question, you might ask 'Where is the evidence that your girlfriend must not pry into your affairs?', whereas an assessment question might be 'Why do you think your girlfriend must not pry into your affairs?', encouraging your client to go more deeply into the reasons why he finds his girlfriend's intrusion personally distressing. To this enquiry, the client may reply 'Because my freedom is being curtailed'. Again, you can ask a disputing question at this point, e.g. 'Why must your freedom not be curtailed?' or, again, you might ask another assessment question, e.g. 'Why is it so important that your freedom must not be curtailed?'. This latter question encourages the client to explore more deeply increasingly relevant aspects of the A.

To complicate matters further, some REBT therapists use what appear to be disputing questions but are really questions designed to help them do inference chaining (Moore, 1983). Thus, instead of asking traditional inference chaining type questions such as 'What is particularly upsetting to you about your girlfriend prying into your affairs?', they ask 'Why must your girlfriend not pry into your affairs?'. When they receive the answer, 'Because my freedom is being curtailed', they ask another question which again seems to be a disputing question, but is really an inference chaining enquiry, e.g. 'Why must your freedom not be curtailed?'.

This use of inference chaining questions which at first sight appear to be disputing questions, is particularly confusing for novice therapists. They think that the therapist is disputing the client's irrational belief, but, really, she is assessing the client's chain of inferences. A solution for this confusion is for novice REBT therapists to discriminate keenly the form of the question from its intent. They need to ask themselves 'Is this question *designed* to challenge a client's irrational belief or *designed* to assess inferential aspects of the A?' If they are successful at doing this, then they will not mix up the two and thereby not confuse themselves or their clients.

> **Key point**
>
> *When asking clients questions, keep clearly in mind the intention of your questions. Keenly discriminate disputing questions and assessment questions.*

62 Encourage your clients to use the principles of overlearning while disputing their irrational beliefs

I stressed earlier in this book (see Point 39) that you need to be repetitive with your clients, while teaching them rational principles. This idea also applies to the disputing process.

The principle of overlearning states that if you go over an idea many times, even more frequently than is perhaps necessary, then you are more likely to retain what you are learning. Thus, encourage your client to challenge her core irrational belief repeatedly, either by using a single proven dispute or by using different types of disputes. Explain to her that the more she is able to do this, the more she will learn how to dispute her beliefs and the more she will remember the outcome of her disputes.

This principle of overlearning also applies to your client acting on her core rational belief. For example, if your client does a shame-attacking exercise every day for six months, she is more likely to effect change than if she does a shame-attacking exercise once a month for six months.

While your client may never completely believe in her core rational belief, given the tendency of human beings to return to well-entrenched irrationalities, if she has overlearned how to dispute her core irrational belief, she will be more likely to dispute it when she identifies it than if she has not overlearned the disputing process. Encourage your client to look upon overlearning through repetition as a form of investment. The more she practices disputing her irrational beliefs now, the greater the benefit she will derive from this later.

> **Key point**
>
> *The more your clients dispute their irrational beliefs, the more they will benefit from this later. So teach them the principle of overlearning and encourage them to apply it.*

Part VI

Dealing with Obstacles to Client Change

63 Assess and deal with obstacles to client changes

There are many potential obstacles to client change that need to be considered when your client is not making progress in REBT. Albert Ellis (1985) has written an entire book on this subject so I will only summarise some of the main points here.

First, when your client is not progressing, ask yourself whether the match between you and your client could be the reason for his lack of progress. You cannot be expected to form productive relationships with all your clients and therefore an honest appraisal of the goodness of fit between you and your client is in order. Some REBT therapists work much more productively with clients who think quickly, and struggle with those who are slower in their thought process. Some therapists have a talent for working with clients who are severely disturbed and have complex problems, while others do much more effective work with clients who are mildly disturbed and have clearly delineated problems. Make an honest inventory of your strengths and weaknesses as an REBT therapist and work on overcoming your weaknesses. In the meantime, you may wish to consider referring your client on to another REBT therapist if you suspect that he or she may work more effectively with that client.

When trying to account for obstacles to client change, consider your client's interpersonal environment. Many clients have the active and on-going support of their significant others who encourage them to enhance their therapy-derived gains. Other clients, however, may be in relationships with people who have an investment in them staying the same. If this is the case, you need to give careful consideration to the advantages and disadvantages of trying to involve these significant others in the therapeutic process: (1) to encourage them to address their own difficulties (say in couples or family therapy); (2) to neutralise their negative impact on your client; or (3) to encourage them to be therapeutic aides if this is possible.

If you cannot involve your client's significant others in the therapeutic process, then you may need to renegotiate your client's goals, particularly if he does not wish to sever his relationship with these other people. If he *does* wish to sever this relationship, you need to support him in this, although obviously this is an important decision which needs to be carefully explored with him. Help him first to overcome his emotional disturbance before you help him to make a sound decision on this issue.

It is important for you to recognise that you, as therapist, may serve as an obstacle to client progress. The effect of therapists' irrational beliefs on the counselling process will be discussed later on in this book (see Point 75), so I will confine myself to a discussion of other hindering therapist variables.

You may prevent client change by adopting an overly optimistic view of the rate of client change. You may be under the misapprehension that REBT is always a fast-acting therapy and not appreciate how difficult your clients may find it to overcome their entrenched problems. This may lead you to put too much pressure on your clients to undertake assignments which they consider overwhelming for them.

You may also obstruct client change by failing to push your clients enough. Here you may form overly warm and cosy therapeutic relationships with them and think that such personal bonds are sufficient to promote client change. You may also have an aversion to the more vigorous aspects of REBT and over compensate by failing to challenge your clients sufficiently.

Another major therapy obstacle to client change is the unskilful practice of REBT. As I often say in my training courses, REBT is an easy therapy to practice unskilfully and it follows that you need to refine and improve your REBT skills by seeking ongoing consultation and supervision.

The final set of obstacles to client change that I wish to discuss here concerns those that emanate from clients themselves. I have deliberately placed this set of factors last to counteract the unfortunate tendency of some therapists to blame clients for their lack of therapeutic change. However, I do think it is also a mistake to exonerate the client completely for non-improvement. Therefore it is important to consider some of the major client obstacles to change which you will commonly encounter. Albert Ellis has long claimed that a philosophy of low frustration tolerance (LFT) in clients is the major obstacle to progress in REBT. This philosophy can interfere with the therapeutic process in a number of different ways. First, due to LFT your client may not remain in therapy for a sufficient length of time for the process to have an impact on him. He may believe that REBT must be a short-term intervention and terminate therapy when he does not make appreciable progress quickly. Second, a philosophy of LFT can interfere with your client's ability to attend to what you say during therapy. Clients who fall into this category may have a limited span of attention and may be easily distracted by relatively unimportant aspects of the counselling process, e.g. the environment in which therapy occurs.

If your client has a philosophy of LFT, he may refuse to do homework assignments or may do them in a half-hearted manner. Research has shown clients who complete self-help assignments in REBT, and other approaches to cognitive behaviour therapy, improve more than clients who fail to complete them (Burns and Nolen-Hoeksema, 1991). Thus, if your client does not do homework assignments, then that remains a significant obstacle to therapeutic progress. However, clients with LFT who do their homework may gain minimal benefit from it. For example, they may do the assignments half-heartedly; they may not give them sufficient time; they may carry them out in an overly intellectual manner and not fully involve themselves in the cognitive, emotive and behavioural aspects of such assignments. The result of such lack of commitment is, unfortunately, lack of progress.

Another significant obstacle to client change concerns the interpersonal problems which your client has with other people and which he may bring to therapy. In particular, client hostility towards you is a potential obstacle to therapeutic progress as this tends to pull a defensive reaction from you: you may either respond with counter-hostility, or you may withdraw and fail to engage the client in a helpful working alliance. At many of his workshops, David Burns has placed a lot of emphasis on this point. He argues that the vast majority of therapists fail to respond therapeutically and empathically when clients act in a hostile manner in therapy. As such, this is an important and unfortunately neglected area of therapist training. Thus, it is very important that you bring such cases to supervision and learn empathic ways of responding to client hostility.

> **Key point**
>
> *Realise that there are many potential obstacles to client change, including poor client–therapist matching; therapist factors, client factors and the negative impact of clients' significant others. Assess these carefully and take remedial action.*

64 Recognise that your clients bring their irrational beliefs to REBT

It is important that you recognise that your client will bring her irrational beliefs (iBs) to REBT and that you try to predict how these beliefs will affect her behaviour in therapy. Do this so that you can take appropriate preventive or remedial action to minimise client resistance. Let me discuss some examples.

A client who has a high need for achievement may well bring this attitude to REBT and become discouraged when she does not achieve good results from therapy, or angry with herself or with you if she fails to understand rational principles.

A client with a high need for approval may become overly sensitive to your communications and become discouraged if you do not show him a lot of warmth and approval. A client with a high need for freedom and autonomy may respond quite negatively to your didactic explanations and directive suggestions about how she might act between sessions. Finally, a client with anger-related iBs may become angry with you when you fall short of perfect professional behaviour.

While it is a mistake to assume that your client will definitely bring her iBs to therapy, it is a good idea to check this out with her. If your client has approval-related iBs, ask her how, if at all, this might affect her relationship with you. If she has achievement-related iBs, ask her how she would cope if she experiences difficulty achieving her therapeutic goals. If you both consider that the client is bringing her iBs to therapy, deal with this in the usual manner using the ABCs of REBT.

> **Key point**
>
> *Client progress can be held up because clients bring their irrational beliefs to the therapeutic process. Try to anticipate how your clients' iBs might affect their behaviour in therapy. Assess and defuse any iBs which hamper your clients' progress.*

65 Elicit and deal with your clients' doubts about REBT

In Point 7, I argued that it was important that you establish and maintain what I called the reflection process where you and your client stand back, reflect and communicate about what you have experienced. As such, this process can be regarded as metatherapy, i.e. a therapeutic discussion about therapeutic work. One important item that you need to discuss during the reflection process is the doubts your client may have about REBT.

It is likely that many clients will have a number of doubts about REBT and its principles. Some may regard REBT as being overly simplistic, others may question the principle of self-acceptance, yet others may wonder about the lack of attention it places on their past and have reservations about the active–directive style of its practitioners, since this style conflicts with common expectations of therapist passivity.

If you do not encourage your client to express his doubts to you, then he will still harbour such doubts and will be heavily influenced by them. If, however, you encourage your client to disclose his doubts to you, then you can discuss these openly with him and correct any misconceptions that he may hold. If you can discuss such issues non-defensively with your client while fully accepting him for having these doubts, then you can serve as a very good role model for dealing with criticism constructively. In addition, when you encourage your client to share his doubts about REBT, he considers that his views are taken seriously, and begins to see himself as an active participant in the therapeutic process and not the passive recipient of rational wisdom.

> **Key point**
>
> *Many of your clients will have doubts about some aspect of REBT. Encourage them to share their doubts and deal with them in a non-defensive manner.*

66 Assess and deal with your clients' misinterpretations of your disputing strategies

Always remember that your disputing interventions serve as activating events for your client during therapy. As such, you need to consider what interpretations and evaluations your client is making about your disputing strategies. If a client misunderstands the meaning behind one of your disputes, then her misunderstanding will have a negative influence on the therapeutic process, particularly if it is unexamined.

To illustrate this phenomenon, I will briefly describe an example. I have a client who is quite unassertive and has difficulty forming relationships with women. He gets particularly lonely at weekends and when he becomes aware of this feeling, he condemns himself for being lonely. My initial therapeutic strategy has been to encourage him to accept himself for being alone so that he does not become depressed. This, I argue, will help him to become active and increase his chances of meeting people over the weekend. However, during one session when I was disputing his self-condemnatory belief, I noticed that my client was becoming quite discouraged. I brought this to his attention and wondered aloud what might be going through his mind as we talked. After some hesitation, he admitted that he thought I was trying to convey to him that he would never get a girlfriend. If I had not become aware of his non-verbal behaviour during the session and encouraged him to share his experience, I would have left unchallenged his incorrect view that I was communicating a vote of no confidence in him. This would have been extraordinarily counter-productive to the self-acceptance work that I was, in fact, trying to do with him.

> **Key point**
>
> *As you dispute your clients' irrational beliefs, assess whether they are misinterpreting what you are trying to accomplish and if so, deal with these misinterpretations in a constructive manner.*

67 Ensure that your clients do not subtly undermine or counteract their new rational beliefs

When your client disputes her irrational beliefs, she can help herself to strengthen her newly developed rational beliefs by acting as if she already believes them. Thus, if your client is working to overcome her dire need for approval, she can counteract this irrational belief by disputing it cognitively and by speaking up and saying unpopular things in public. However, be aware that your client can subtly undermine her newly emerging rational beliefs by acting as if she still believed her more entrenched irrational beliefs. Thus, it will be difficult for your client, in the example quoted above, to achieve real gains in therapy if she cognitively disputed her need for approval, but continued to keep quiet in social situations.

A clear example of where a client can undermine his progress in this way occurred with a client of mine who wanted to overcome his addiction to visiting prostitutes. He claimed that although he tried to dispute his irrational belief 'I must have sexual satisfaction quickly', he did not believe his dispute. It transpired that he carried out his disputing assignment while walking towards the local brothel! By doing so, he was subtly undermining his disputes because he was acting as if he believed that he had to have his sexual desires fulfilled immediately.

Clients with panic disorder frequently undermine their new rational beliefs in subtle ways. Such clients can, while showing themselves that they can stand their strong feelings of anxiety, act in subtle ways to reduce their anxiety. For example, they may sit down when they think that they might pass out, or they may distract themselves from their symptoms as a way of avoiding their anxious feelings. These subtle manoeuvres serve unwittingly to reinforce these clients' irrational belief that they cannot tolerate intense anxiety since they act as if they cannot tolerate it.

> **Key point**
>
> *You will need to carry out a detailed assessment of the subtle ways that clients act to avoid, and thereby reinforce, their fears. If you do not do so, your clients will undermine the beneficial effects of cognitive disputing.*

Part VII

Creativity

68 Make judicious use of referrals

It may seem strange to begin this section on creativity in REBT by advocating the use of referrals. However, I agree with Arnold Lazarus (see Dryden, 1991) who argues that effecting suitable referrals is an important skill in the repertoire of all therapists.

The following are examples of situations in which you might refer a client.

1. When your client needs specialist help from another REBT therapist who has expertise in that particular area. Although REBT is a general approach to psychotherapy, different REBT therapists have different areas of expertise. Thus, you might try to help a client who is depressed because she has just lost her young son through sudden infant death syndrome or you may usefully refer her to another REBT therapist who specialises in this area (Schneiman, 1993). This REBT therapist may have a fuller understanding of client reactions to this syndrome and may appreciate better the nuances of the therapeutic technique that needs to be used with such clients.
2. When a client seeks REBT, but you consider that she may form a stronger working alliance with one of your colleagues, given the personality and temperamental characteristics of the client, yourself and the colleague to whom you wish to make the referral.
3. When the client, in your opinion, may be better helped by a therapist from a different school of therapy. This may be because the client's problem is better approached by a therapist from a different orientation, or because the client's therapeutic preferences are more likely to be met by a therapist of a different persuasion. For example, a client may have tension headaches which require biofeedback training, which you as an REBT therapist may not be competent to practise. In this situation you may wish to refer the client to a biofeedback expert. If the biofeedback therapist also has skills in REBT, then so much the better. If not, you may both work concurrently or consecutively with the client.
4. When a client articulates a preference for a different type of psychotherapy. This is more difficult to deal with, since the client may be harbouring certain misconceptions about REBT and have certain positive, but unrealistic expectations about the benefits of another type of therapy. In this case, you would want to initiate a full and frank discussion about the client's expectations of therapy, in general, and understanding of REBT, in particular; at the end of this discussion you might offer the client a short trial period of REBT. However, it is better to refer some clients to a therapist from a different orientation than to try to use REBT when they do not want it. While REBT is an effective approach to psychotherapy, guard against

a dogmatic conviction that it is right for everybody, and the equally dogmatic view that you are the most suitable therapist for all clients.

> **Key point**
>
> *Consider referring some clients to your REBT colleagues or to non-REBT therapists.*

69 Be flexible in your use of therapy sessions

A book written for the general public called *Same Time Next Week?* (Neimark, 1981) warned against the dangers of the weekly fix of psychotherapy where clients attend psychotherapy at the same time every week, for the same duration every week, no doubt discussing the same problems every week! To guard against this timeless nature of on-going therapy, it is important that you are flexible in your use of therapy sessions. I have already recommended (in Point 41) increasing the length of time between therapy sessions as you approach the end of REBT.

You also need to be flexible in the duration of your therapy sessions. Albert Ellis offers two types of therapy sessions for individual patients: half-hour sessions and one-hour sessions. I have listened to many of these sessions and it seems to me that Ellis works harder and faster in the half-hour sessions than he does in the one-hour sessions. The famous or infamous 50-minute hour was invented for the benefit of therapists rather than for the benefit of clients in that it enabled therapists to have a short (10 minute) break between sessions.

However, you will find that certain clients cannot make use of a 50-minute therapy session. Such clients may have low IQ or a limited attention span and will just become confused if you see them for 50 minutes. With such clients, experiment with varying the length of therapy sessions; offer some of them 20 minutes, in which time you may just cover one point with them. However, this investment of a short period of time pays off because the client is more likely to remember that one point than if several points were discussed in a 50-minute period.

Conversely, you may need to spend longer than 50 minutes with other clients. This is certainly true with clients who live out of town and travel long distances for a therapy session. Being one of the few REBT therapists in Britain, I have had a lot of experience of seeing clients for one- or two-off sessions given the fact that they live a long way from London where I practise. In these circumstances, I may see such clients for a two-hour period or, exceptionally, for a three-hour period in which we discuss a variety of their problems. I routinely tape-record these sessions and give them a copy of the audiotapes for later review.

One way of encouraging client independence is to increase the time interval between therapy sessions. Raymond DiGiuseppe has suggested that therapy sessions are scheduled no more frequently than a client's emotional upsets. Thus, if your client is upset every seven days, then a weekly session will probably suffice. However, if she is upset every eight days, then fortnightly sessions might be preferable. While I think it is a helpful suggestion, I do not think that DiGiuseppe would argue that clients who are upset every day need to be seen every day!

Other flexible uses of therapy include having telephone sessions and responding to client letters by writing to them. On a recent trip to America, my good friend and colleague Richard Wessler told me about a therapy he was conducting by letter with a man from Greece. While therapy through the mail should of course not replace face-to-face therapy, it certainly can be helpful as numerous agony aunts and uncles will testify.

When you are considering flexible modifications to the use of therapy sessions, these modifications need to be based upon a clear rationale. This should be discussed with the client, and she needs to agree to the modification.

> **Key point**
>
> *Be prepared to be flexible in your use of therapy sessions, modifying their duration and form. Elicit agreement from your clients whenever you wish to deviate from the standard, face-to-face 50-minute hour.*

70 Use techniques from other therapeutic approaches, but in a manner consistent with REBT theory

As early as 1962, Ellis advocated using techniques from other therapeutic approaches, but in ways which are consistent with REBT theory. I consider REBT to be a good example of what I call theoretically consistent eclecticism (Dryden, 1987). Here, you use REBT theory to formulate a therapeutic strategy and you are free to use REBT techniques or techniques spawned from other therapies when you implement the strategy. As Arnold Lazarus argues (see Dryden, 1991), when you use a technique that originates from a different approach to therapy, you are not obliged to buy into the theoretical principles which gave birth to the technique in question. Thus, when you use a two-chair technique that was originally developed by gestalt therapists, you are not making the same assumptions that they make; rather, you are using the technique to achieve a goal that is consistent with REBT theory. When a gestalt therapist uses two-chair work, one of her major purposes is to help her client resolve splits in psychological functioning. When an REBT therapist uses chair-work, it may be to encourage the client to practise weakening an irrational belief and strengthening a rational belief.

When you borrow techniques from other therapeutic approaches, it is important that you give careful thought to possible unintended consequences. For example, cathartic techniques may well help your client to identify her feelings at point C in the ABC framework, but such techniques may also encourage her to strengthen the irrational belief which underpins her feelings.

So far, I have discussed borrowing techniques from other therapeutic approaches to implement clinical strategies consistent with REBT theory. It is possible, however, to borrow techniques or ways of working from other therapeutic approaches which improve the structure of REBT therapy sessions. Thus, I often make problem lists with clients and set session agendas with them, since I believe that doing so encourages both of us to use time effectively in therapy. Both of these methods, I should add, are derived from Beck's cognitive therapy (compare Beck et al., 1979).

> **Key point**
>
> *REBT is a theoretically consistent form of eclectic therapy. As such, it encourages you to borrow techniques and working practices from other therapeutic approaches, but in a manner consistent with REBT theory.*

71 Vary the medium, but not the message

In point 39, I mentioned the importance of being repetitive in your communication of rational principles. I suggested that you either teach a rational principle repetitively in the same way, or that you should use different ways of communicating the same message. Here I will elaborate on the latter point and illustrate what I mean by it.

As discussed in point 53, you can use different styles in disputing your client's irrational beliefs (i.e. didactic, socratic, metaphorical, humorous and enactive). Let us see how this principle applies when you show your client the value of self-acceptance. You can didactically explain the concept to your client. Second, you can engage her in a socratic dialogue by asking pertinent questions until she has grasped the point. Third, you can tell your client a story to illustrate the importance of not giving people a global rating. For example, Wessler and Wessler (1980) discuss the case of Nathan Leopold who, as a teenager, killed a young boy for a thrill, was sent to prison for a long sentence, educated himself while he was serving his sentence, trained to be a social worker on his release and did excellent work with disadvantaged groups. The question they ask is: 'How do we rate Nathan Leopold? Is he a good person or a bad person?'. The answer is neither. He is a fallible human being, who once did a very bad thing for which he was punished but later did many good deeds.

A humorous way of communicating the principle of self-acceptance is to describe the game of rational and irrational tennis. An example of irrational tennis is this: 'I hit a bad shot, therefore I am a bad person – I hit a good shot, therefore I am a good person'. An example of rational tennis is this: 'I hit a bad shot, therefore I am a fallible person – I hit a good shot, therefore I am a fallible person'.

An example of using an enactive technique to teach self-acceptance is asking your client to give you various traits, behaviours and different aspects of himself which you write down on yellow 'post-it' notes. You stick these on different parts of the client's body until he is covered with notes from head to foot. The question you then ask is: can your client be given a single rating which completely accounts for him? The answer is no, he is too complex to be given such a rating.

You can combine an enactive method with a humorous technique by throwing a glass of water over yourself and asking your client: 'Was that a silly thing to do?' to which the client frequently replies, 'Yes'. You then ask him: 'Does that therefore make me a silly person?' to which, hopefully, the client responds, 'No'!

In addition, you can use other media to demonstrate the value of self-acceptance. For example, consider Figure 4 which illustrates what it takes to be a good person (i.e. have only good traits, behaviours etc.), a bad person (have only bad traits, behaviours etc.), a fallible person (have a mixture of good, bad and neutral traits, behaviours etc.). Frequently, a visual display such as this communicates more than a 1000-word explanation of the value of self-acceptance.

Here, as elsewhere, you are only limited by your therapeutic imagination!

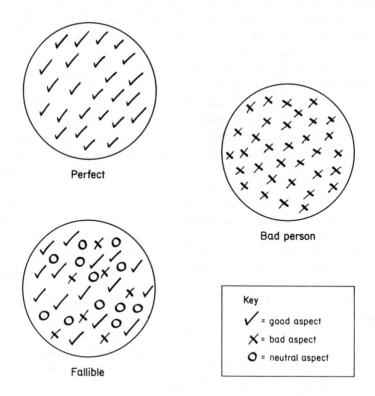

Figure 4 Viewing the self as fallible.

> **Key point**
>
> *Realise that you can teach a rational principle, such as the value of self-acceptance, in many different ways. So, use your imagination and vary the medium, but not the message.*

72 Be vivid in your interventions, but avoid being too vivid

In the early 1980s, I wrote of the importance of doing REBT in a vivid way (Dryden, 1986). By this, I meant making your interventions memorable so that your client can readily remember the rational principles which you are teaching her. Since REBT is an educational approach to psychotherapy, your client will be more likely to use rational principles in her life if she is able to remember them. Vivid methods are effective because they stimulate your client's imagination and more fully engage your client's emotions.

In Point 53, I argued that it is important for you to check that your client understands the metaphors, stories, anecdotes, parables and aphorisms that you use. Your client can easily misinterpret the meaning of these interventions since they convey rational principles in indirect ways. To ascertain that your client has understood the meaning, you need to ask your client to share her understanding of the point you are trying to make. The same is true when you use vivid interventions, particularly when the rational principle that you are attempting to teach is implicit in the intervention. You should also note that some of your clients will not respond well to vivid interventions since they believe that as a therapist, you should be serious. This conflicts with your behaviour when you use vivid interventions which are humorous and dramatic in nature. It is important to gauge your client's reactions to your use of these methods by referring this issue to the reflection process.

In my original writings on what I called vivid REBT, I cautioned therapists about the indiscriminate overuse of vivid methods. I would like to underscore this point here since the judicious use of a single vivid intervention in a session may have far greater impact on your client than the continuous use of such methods in the same session. Indeed, when you use a lot of vivid methods, your client may well become confused or dazzled and thereby forget the principles which the vivid interventions were meant to illustrate. Never forget that vivid methods in REBT are instrumental: their purpose is to highlight a rational principle so that it is likely to be remembered. You should rarely use vivid therapeutic methods in REBT as an end in themselves.

> **Key point**
>
> *Make judicious use of vivid methods in REBT to help your clients remember and apply rational principles. Guard against overusing such methods.*

73 Create new REBT techniques

In my experience, the most effective REBT practitioners are those who are creative and continually discover new techniques. This creative process depends on the ability to think laterally and to use everyday occurrences as stimuli to creative thinking.

Let me give a personal example of this creative process in action. About a year ago, I was strolling in a shopping centre when I passed a shop that had a variety of novelty products on sale, including large red and yellow plastic swords. I did not immediately think of how these could be used in REBT, but after walking along the road for a further 25 yards, an idea came to me. I thought of the following dramatic way in which I could use the swords to help my clients to strengthen their rational beliefs and weaken their irrational beliefs. Once I have disputed my client's irrationalities, I bring out the swords and hand the client the red sword (*r* stands for *r*ational) and I take the yellow sword (*y* stands for irrational; unfortunately, they had no swords in *i*ndigo!). I then explain to my client that we are going to engage in a game of rational sword fencing. My task is to use my irrational sword to disarm my client's rational sword and win the fight, and the client's task is to vanquish my irrational sword with her rational one. I instruct my client to be as vigorous as possible in stating her rational belief and hitting my sword. I then attack her rational argument by stating the contrary irrational belief while hitting her sword. This technique works particularly well in group therapy where the group members have a good relationship with one another and where they do not consider the use of this method patronising or belittling.

> **Key point**
>
> *Let your mind drift and use the creative aspects of your imagination to invent new REBT techniques.*

74 Capitalise on your clients' pre-therapy experiences of personal change

Do not forget that before seeking therapeutic help, your client will have had quite a few experiences of personal change. In order to capitalise on these pre-therapy change experiences, you need to identify them. Ask your client about times in his life when he has changed an unhealthy attitude, a self-defeating behaviour or a disturbed emotion. Do this at the beginning of therapy or after you have actually disputed his irrational beliefs. Devote some time to understanding what it was that the client did to bring about this change and, if this is broadly consistent with REBT theory, show him that he can use himself as a role model for change on the problem you are discussing. Examples of how clients have effected change by their own efforts include: going for a long walk to think things through, talking to sensible members of the family and putting into practice their advice, thinking of how somebody healthy would handle a situation and then using that person as a role model and writing out the pro's and con's of a particular piece of behaviour etc. Integrate these change processes with REBT methods: such a combination can be quite powerful. However, guard against using a client's successful self-change methods when these may prevent him from achieving elegant philosophical change.

Jerome Frank has argued that one of the major curative factors of psychotherapy is that it engenders hope (Frank & Frank, 1991). Helping your client see that he has been successful in dealing with past emotional problems and that he can regard himself as an inspiring but realistic role model, can be a powerful way of engendering hope in your client.

Key point

Discover and capitalise on your clients' pre-therapy experiences of personal change. Integrate these with REBT methods, but guard against using any of their change experiences which conflict with philosophical change.

Part VIII

Develop Yourself both Personally and Professionally

75 Identify and dispute your own irrational beliefs about your clients and the process of therapy

In Point 63, I argued that therapist factors are an important source of client resistance. Here I want to consider one such factor: the irrational beliefs that you as an REBT therapist might hold about your clients in the therapeutic process. Ellis (1985) has outlined the following therapist irrational beliefs that interfere with the effective practice of REBT.

1. I *have to* be successful with all my clients practically all the time.
2. I *must* be an outstanding therapist, clearly better than other therapists I know or hear about.
3. I *have to* be greatly respected and loved by all my clients.
4. Since I am doing my best and working so hard as a therapist, my clients *should* be equally hardworking and responsible, *should* listen to me carefully, and *should* always push themselves to change.
5. Because I am a person in my own right, I *must* be able to enjoy myself during therapy sessions and to use the sessions to solve my personal problems as much as to help clients with their difficulties.

In my experience, it is difficult for REBT therapists to acknowledge that they hold such attitudes. This may be compounded by an additional irrational belief that many REBT therapists hold: 'Now that I am a REBT therapist, I must not be irrational, particularly about therapy'. If you can accept yourself as a fallible human being who may well have irrational beliefs which become apparent inside as well as outside therapy, you can then take the next step, to monitor your feelings and behaviour, and use these as a guide to the detection of your therapy-related irrational beliefs. One factor that may stop you from doing this is an additional irrational belief: 'I must not experience unhealthy negative emotions, particularly when I am doing REBT'. If you can accept yourself for having such feelings in therapy, you may watch for the following signs that you may be holding irrational beliefs about your clients or the process of therapy:

1. If you find yourself making blaming and condemning remarks about your clients, you may be holding a low frustration tolerance (LFT)-related irrational belief which leads to anger, or you may be experiencing defensive anger in response to a perceived threat to your self-esteem.
2. If you find yourself using scare tactics with your clients, this may

well indicate that: (a) you may be demanding that your clients prove, by their progress, what a great therapist and therefore worthwhile person you are; or (b) you have an LFT-related belief about how quickly therapy must proceed.
3. When you catch yourself making judgmental remarks about your clients or having judgement-related angry feelings towards them, this may indicate that you are intolerant of your clients' weaknesses or that you have LFT-related impatience.
4. When you are unrealistic and offer your clients false hopes about therapy, this is frequently a sign that you wish to bolster your threatened ego by showing yourself what a great therapist you are in what you can achieve, or that you have an underlying need for your clients' approval.
5. If you find yourself getting caught in argumentative power struggles with your clients, then this may indicate that you have a need to be right or to be seen to be right by your clients, or that you are intolerant of your clients' negative views about rational principles and the process of REBT.

When you discover one or more of these irrational beliefs, accept yourself for holding them and vigorously dispute them. For a more detailed discussion of these and other attitudinal errors made by REBT therapists, consult Walen, DiGiuseppe and Dryden (1992).

> **Key point**
>
> *Honestly acknowledge your therapy-related irrational beliefs, accept yourself for holding them and dispute them vigorously.*

76 Beware the neurotic agreement

In an important early, but sadly neglected paper, Paul Hauck (1966) discussed what he called the neurotic agreement in psychotherapy. By this, he referred to the situation where you share your client's irrational beliefs. Thus, if your client is talking about how horrible it would be to lose his job and you also believe that it would be horrible to lose your job, then it will be difficult for you to do effective REBT with the client on this issue.

A clue to the existence of a neurotic agreement in psychotherapy is that your normally skilful practice of REBT breaks down. You may subtly change the subject when your client discusses material that you find disturbing, or you may be quite tentative when the time comes to dispute your client's irrational beliefs. Occasionally, when you share your client's irrational beliefs, you may attack these beliefs too vigorously. This may well be a form of projection or you may underlyingly hate yourself for holding such beliefs and thereby hate the client for reminding you of your own unacceptable irrationality.

The following are ways that you can identify neurotic agreements in psychotherapy.

1. Pay attention to your disturbed feelings or look for signs that you may be ashamed of having such feelings, e.g. you may find yourself engaging in various defensive manoeuvres to protect yourself from experiencing these feelings.
2. Listen to audiotapes of your therapy sessions when you suspect the presence of a neurotic agreement. Here, pay particular attention to your behaviour which may be defensive in nature. Once you recognise such defensive behaviour, it is easier to ask yourself what you are defending yourself against. Since doing this for yourself may be difficult, seek on-going supervision, even if you are a seasoned REBT therapist (see Point 77).

Once you have identified a neurotic agreement and you have accepted yourself for having an irrational belief which is similar to that of your client, use your REBT skills with yourself. If you reach this stage, then you will be able to do this; the greater difficulty lies in acknowledging that you neurotically agree with your client's irrational belief.

> **Key point**
>
> *Look for signs that you neurotically agree with your clients' irrational beliefs. Accept yourself for sharing your clients' irrationalities and dispute your own irrational beliefs.*

77 Seek regular supervision

I am an accredited counsellor with the British Association for Counselling. In order to maintain my accredited status, I have to prove that I am in on-going supervision. The minimum amount of on-going supervision has been set at 1.5 hours per month in individual supervision and an equivalent period if one is attending group supervision.

From what I know of the American scene, such on-going supervision is not generally required as a pre-condition for professional membership. This is a pity, since no matter how experienced you are, you always have blind spots and it often takes a fresh pair of ears to help you identify them.

Since REBT therapists value the use of audio recordings of therapy sessions, as they highlight what is actually going on between therapist and client, supervision is often based on such tapes (which are, of course, only used with the client's expressed permission). However, a broader discussion of cases where treatment planning is reviewed is also extremely useful.

While novice REBT therapists are likely to seek supervision from more experienced colleagues, experienced REBT therapists are more likely to benefit from peer supervision, where two colleagues of equal standing supervise each other's work. Ruth Wessler and I had probably the longest-standing REBT peer supervisory arrangement, since for 10 years we sent each other tapes of our therapy sessions for supervision.

In order to get the most out of supervision, it is important that you prepare for it. Review a particular session and cue specific portions of the tape that you wish to play to your supervisor. This is important since, as a supervisor, I know how frustrating it is to supervise a tape when the supervisee has not listened to it before the supervision session. Such behaviour may be a function of the supervisee's low frustration tolerance or it may be a defensive manoeuvre to throw the supervisor off the scent. If the latter is the case, it may be an indication that the supervisee has irrational beliefs about needing the approval of his supervisor or about being seen to be competent. This can be gently explored by the supervisor as long as supervision does not become personal therapy.

> **Key point**
>
> *Commit yourself to regular, on-going supervision so that you can enhance your skilful practice of REBT.*

78 Transcribe therapy sessions periodically and evaluate each of your interventions

In addition to seeking supervision, I recommend that you engage in self-supervision. This can take the form of listening to tapes of your therapy sessions while using a self-supervision inventory such as the one found in the appendix of Wessler and Wessler (1980).

Additionally, I have found it helpful periodically to transcribe a randomly selected REBT session and to evaluate each of my responses in terms of my intentions and skill level. I pay particular attention to how

I could have phrased my responses more skilfully. This intense microanalysis of a therapy session is time consuming and cannot be done regularly. However, it reveals important information about skills deficits, lacunae, poorly considered strategies etc. Whenever I undertake this analysis, it is quite a humbling experience. However, I occasionally recognise that I am not such a bad REBT therapist after all! Such transcripts can also be used as a basis for supervision from a more experienced REBT colleague.

It is also useful to study transcripts of experienced REBT therapists. Fortunately, we have not been reticent about publishing session transcripts and I direct the reader to the transcribed sessions in *Growth through Reason* (Ellis, 1971) and in *Daring to be Myself* (Dryden and Yankura, 1992). The latter text contains full transcripts of an entire brief therapy with on-going commentary.

> **Key point**
>
> *Periodically, transcribe your therapy sessions and evaluate the skilfulness of your interventions, the suitability of your interventions and the helpfulness of your strategies.*

79 Use REBT in your own life

It is not known to what extent REBT therapists use REBT in their own lives, but it would be strange if they did not do so to some degree. Indeed, it is one good way of keeping your own REBT therapy skills well-honed.

I have used REBT to cope with an extended period of unemployment in the mid 1980s as well as with my on-going problem of anger. In this latter respect, I believe I have an inherited tendency towards anger and, while I cannot do anything about ridding myself of that, I have learned to apply my REBT skills as soon as I recognise that I am beginning to make myself angry, so that I do not perpetuate my angry feelings.

I used skills similar to those advocated by REBT earlier in my life to help me overcome my anxiety about speaking in public. In fact, I believe I became an REBT therapist because there was a high degree of congruence between my natural emotional problem-solving style and that advocated by REBT.

I would also recommend that all REBT therapists have therapy with a seasoned REBT professional (1) to address blind spots which they may not be able to identify on their own; (2) to help overcome problems that they have not been able to overcome on their own through

REBT self-therapy methods; and (3) to see how it feels to be a client in the REBT process.

In the course of my many discussions with Albert Ellis over the years which have centred mainly on points of theory and practice, I have occasionally brought up a number of personal issues and have been helped through my discussions with him. Incidentally, on occasion, I have had to urge him to slow down because he has a very fast mind and can quickly see what I am telling myself to disturb myself. Even though I know REBT theory and practice very well, I find that I cannot keep up with his quickfire and accurate interventions!

> **Key point**
>
> Use REBT in your own life as much as you can. Also, consider seeking personal therapy from an experienced REBT therapist.

80 Develop your own style in therapy and in life

It is perhaps quite understandable that novice REBT therapists try to model themselves after Albert Ellis before developing their own more authentic therapeutic style. There are many effective REBT styles and it is worthwhile to study carefully tapes in the Institute for Rational–Emotive Therapy's professional tape library (on sale from IRET, 45 East 65th Street, New York, NY 10021, USA).

More serious, however, is the tendency amongst some REBT therapists to try to model themselves after Ellis's work pattern. Albert Ellis has a very heavy work schedule which he seems to enjoy and to which he seems to be temperamentally suited. It is a serious error and potentially unhealthy for therapists who have a different temperament and who have different priorities in life to try to emulate Ellis on this point. I end this book, therefore, by encouraging you to know yourself, know your temperament, know your interests and preferred work patterns and to look after yourself. In particular, take short breaks between therapy sessions, do not neglect your physical and mental well-being and do not neglect to nurture and be nurtured by your loved ones.

It may seem strange to end a book on REBT in this way: after all, REBT has been portrayed as a tough-minded approach to therapy in a tender-minded profession (Weinrach, 1994). However, since REBT seeks to integrate different elements of healthy human functioning into its broadly-based therapeutic approach, there is no reason why you cannot also take a tender minded attitude towards yourself!

Develop yourself both personally and professionally

> **Key points**
>
> *Do not try to emulate Albert Ellis's style of therapy or work pattern unless you are suited to these styles. Be yourself and look after yourself in therapy and in life.*

References

Beck, A.T., Rush, A.J., Shaw, B.F. and Emery, G. (1979). *Cognitive Therapy of Depression*. New York: Guilford.

Bordin, E.S. (1979). The generalisability of the psychoanalytic concept of the working alliance. *Psychotherapy: Theory, Research and Practice* 16, 252–260.

Budman, S.H. and Gurman, A.S. (1988). *Theory and Practice of Brief Therapy*. New York: Guilford.

Burns, D.D. (1980). *Feeling Good: The New Mood Therapy*. New York: Morrow.

Burns, D.D. and Nolen-Hoeksema, S. (1991). Coping styles, homework assignments, and the effectiveness of cognitive–behavioral therapy. *Journal of Consulting and Clinical Psychology* 59, 305–311.

Burns, D.D. and Nolen-Hoeksema, S. (1992). Therapeutic empathy and recovery from depression in cognitive–behavioral therapy: A structural equation model. *Journal of Consulting and Clinical Psychology* 60, 441–449.

DiGiuseppe, R. (1991). Comprehensive cognitive disputing in rational-emotive therapy. In: M. Bernard (Ed.), *Using Rational-Emotive Therapy Effectively*. New York: Plenum.

Dryden, W. (1979). Past messages and disputations: The client and significant others. *Rational Living* 14(1), 26–28.

Dryden, W. (1984). Therapeutic arenas. In: W. Dryden (Ed.), *Individual Therapy in Britain*. London: Harper and Row.

Dryden, W. (1985). Challenging, but not overwhelming: A compromise in negotiating homework assignments. *British Journal of Cognitive Psychotherapy* 3(1), 77–80.

Dryden, W. (1986). Vivid methods in rational–emotive therapy. In: A. Ellis and R. Grieger (Eds), *Handbook of Rational–Emotive Therapy*, volume 2. New York: Springer.

Dryden, W. (1987). *Current Issues in Rational–Emotive Therapy*. Beckenham: Croom Helm.

Dryden, W. (1989a). The use of chaining in rational–emotive therapy. *Journal of Rational–Emotive and Cognitive Behavior Therapy* 7(2), 59–66.

Dryden, W. (Ed.) (1989b). *Howard Young – Rational Therapist: Seminal papers in rational–emotive therapy*. Loughton, Essex: Gale Centre Publications.

Dryden, W. (1990a). *Rational–Emotive Counselling in Action*. London: Sage.

Dryden, W. (Ed.) (1990b). *The Essential Albert Ellis*. New York: Springer.

Dryden, W. (1991). *A Dialogue with Arnold Lazarus: 'It depends'*. Buckingham: Open University Press.

Dryden, W. (Ed.) (1992). *Hard-earned Lessons from Counselling in Action*. London: Sage.

Dryden, W. and DiGiuseppe, R. (1990). *A Primer on Rational–Emotive Therapy*. Champaign, IL: Research Press.

Dryden, W., Ferguson, J. and McTeague, S. (1989). Beliefs and inferences – a test of a rational–emotive hypothesis: 2. On the prospect of seeing a spider. *Psychological Reports* 64, 115–123.

Dryden, W. and Yankura, J. (1992). *Daring to be Myself: A Case of Rational–Emotive Therapy*. Buckingham: Open University Press.

Ellis, A. (1971). *Growth through Reason*. North Hollywood, CA: Wilshire Books.

Ellis, A. (1985). *Overcoming Resistance: Rational–Emotive Therapy with Difficult Patients*. New York: Springer.

Ellis, A. (1989). Ineffective consumerism in the cognitive-behavioural therapies and in general psychotherapy. In: W. Dryden and P. Trower (Eds), *Cognitive Psychotherapy: Stasis and Change*. London: Cassell.

Ellis, A. (1991). The revised ABC's of rational–emotive therapy. *Journal of Rational–Emotive and Cognitive Behavior Therapy* 9, 139–172.

Frank, J.D. and Frank, J.B. (1991). *Persuasion and Healing*, 3rd edn. Baltimore, MD: Johns Hopkins University Press.

Grieger, R. (1989). A client's guide to rational-emotive therapy (RET). In: W. Dryden and P. Trower (Eds), *Cognitive Psychotherapy: Stasis and Change*. London: Cassell.

Hauck, P. (1966). The neurotic agreement in psychotherapy. *Rational Living* 1(1), 32–35.

Jeffers, S. (1987). *Feel the Fear: and Do It Anyway*. London: Century Hutchinson.

Kopp, S. (1977). *Back to One*. Palo Alto, CA: Science and Behavior Books.

Lazarus, A.A. (1984). *In the Mind's Eye*. New York: Guilford Press.

Lazarus, A.A. and Lazarus, C.N. (1991). *Multimodal Life History Inventory*. Champaign, IL: Research Press.

Maultsby, M.C. Jr (1984). *Rational Behavior Therapy*. Englewood Cliffs, NJ: Prentice-Hall.

Moore, R. (1983). Inference as 'A' in RET. *British Journal of Cognitive Psychotherapy* 1(2), 17–23.

Neimark, P. (1981). *Same Time Next Week? How To Leave Your Therapist*. Westport, CT: Arlington House.

Safran, J.D. (1993). The therapeutic alliance rupture as a transtheoretical phenomenon: Definitional and conceptual issues. *Journal of Psychotherapy Integration* 3, 33–49.

Schneiman, R.S. (1993). RET and sudden infant death syndrome. In: W. Dryden and L. Hill (Eds), *Innovations in Rational-Emotive Therapy*. Newbury Park, CA: Sage.

Walen, S.R., DiGiuseppe, R. and Dryden, W. (1992). *A Practitioner's Guide to Rational-Emotive Therapy*, 2nd edn. New York: Oxford University Press.

Weinrach, S.G. (1994). A tough-minded therapy for a tender-minded profession: An irrational field confronts a rational approach. *Journal of Counseling and Development* (in press).

Wessler, R.A. and Wessler, R.L. (1980). *The Principles and Practice of Rational-Emotive Therapy*. San Francisco, CA: Jossey-Bass.

Young, H.S. (1974). *A Rational Counseling Primer*. New York: Institute for Rational–Emotive Therapy.

Index

ABC form, 69–70
ABC model, 26
abuse, 57–58
acceptance
    principle of self-, 119–120
    versus resignation, 32–33
activating events, 41–42, 46
    assessment of, 50–52
    assuming to be true, 85–86
    interpretation of, 30–32
    major new, 47
agenda-setting, 39, 40, 43
anticipatory socialisation practices, 22–23
anxiety
    versus concern, 13
    disorders, 66
approval
    clients' need for, 59
arenas *see* therapeutic arenas
A's *see* activating events
assessment, 40–41
    of A's, 50–52
    for client change, 58
    versus disputing questions, 101–102
    of fear reinforcement, 112
    of obstacles to change, 107–109
    specificity in, 46
assignments *see* homework assignments
audio recordings *see* tape-recording of sessions
avoidant behaviour, 53
awfulising beliefs, 27, 86
    disputing of, 95–96

Beck, A.T., 12, 118
beliefs, 25–26
    awfulising, 27, 86
    condemnatory, 86
    rational versus irrational, 27–28
    self-downing, 27
bibliotherapy, 10
bond domain, 3–4
    varying the bond, 4–6
borderline disturbances, 12
Bordin, Ed, 3
Budman, S.H., 61
Burns, D., 12, 52, 73, 108, 109

case formulations, 53
challenge, 11
'challenging but not overwhelming', 11
change *see* client change, philosophical change
client change
    assessment for, 58
    commitment to, 15
    dealing with obstacles to, 107–112
    encouraging, 65–81
    pre-therapy, 122–123
    reinforcement of, 59
client doubts about REBT, 110–111
client hostility, 109
client responses
    evaluation of, 49
client understanding
    checking of, 9
cognitive therapy, 118
cognitive–emotive dissonance, 98
collaborative empiricism, 7
commitment to change
    clients', 15

coping criterion, 47–48
core irrational beliefs, 52–54
couple therapy, 17
creativity, 115–123
 therapeutic, 61
crises
 clients', 47

defensiveness of therapists, 129
dependency, 53
DiGiuseppe, Raymond, 45, 47, 57, 85, 88–90, 100, 117
directiveness of therapist, 8
disputing, 85–103
 versus assessment questions, 101–102
 and clients' goals, 87–88
 comprehensiveness in, 88–90
 coping model of, 97–98
 didactic, 89
 enactive, 90
 the 'friend dispute', 94–95
 humorous, 89–90
 level of abstraction and, 90
 mastery model of, 97–98
 meaningful, 91
 metaphorical, 89
 misinterpretations of, 111
 one irrational belief only, 86
 others' irrational beliefs, 99–100
 persistent, 92
 pragmatic, 87–88
 socratic, 88–89
 the 'terrorist dispute', 95–96
 vigorous, 92
disturbance *see* emotional disturbance
downward arrow technique, 52
Dryden, W., 11, 12, 16, 17, 31, 41, 45, 47, 57, 69, 75, 85, 90, 91, 92, 100, 115, 117, 118, 131

eclecticism
 theoretically consistent, 117–118
Edelstein, Michael, 91
educational issues, 21–36
Ellis, Albert, 4, 8, 14, 27, 30, 39, 59, 86, 89, 92, 107, 116, 117, 127, 131, 132
emotional disturbance
 dealing with, 29–30
emotional responsibility
 teaching of, 25–26

emotions *see* negative emotions
eye contact, 55

family therapy, 17–18
feeling words
 use of, 13
Ferguson, J., 31
fifty-minute hour, 116
first principles
 returning to, 60–61
formality
 degree of therapist, 4–5
Frank, J.B., 123
Frank, J.D., 123

generalisation of learning, 80–81
goal domain, 3
 disturbance versus self-fulfilment, 14
goal-directed stance, 14–15
grief, 56–57
Grieger, Russ, 23
group therapy, 18
Gurman, A.S., 61

Hauck, Paul, 74, 128
histrionic personality, 40
homework assignments, 11, 71, 108–109
 apprehension about, 79
 behavioural, 74–75, 78–79
 checking of, 77–80
 daily self-help, 76–77
 data-collection, 77–78
 educational, 78
 failure to do, 59
 imagery, 74, 78
 negotiation of, 73–76
 non-completion of, 75–76
 ordering of, 74–75
 problem list in, 44
hope, 123
hostility
 client, 109
humour
 in disputing, 89–90
 songs, 90
 therapist, 5–6, 119

imagery
 assignments, 74, 78
 time-tripping, 93
individual therapy, 17

Index

inferential chain, 51, 52, 102
influence base of therapist, 6–7
information-gathering strategies, 40–42
interventions
    evaluation of, 130–131
    vividness in, 120–121
irrational beliefs
    core, 52–54
    disputing one only, 86–87
    disputing of others', 99–100
    effect of on A, 30–32
    hidden, 54–55
    versus rational beliefs, 27–28
    in the therapeutic process, 110
    therapist insensitivity and, 57–58
    of therapists, 127–128
irrationality
    time-limited, 55–57, 93
    see also irrational beliefs

Jeffers, Susan, 98

Kopp, Sheldon, 60–61

language
    use of a common, 12–13
Lazarus, A.A., 41, 93, 115, 118
Lazarus, C.N., 41
learning
    client responsibility for, 9–10
    facilitating clients', 9–10
    generalisation of, 80–81
    see also overlearning
low frustration tolerance, 27, 77, 86
    and homework assignments, 75
    as obstacle to change, 108–109

McTeague, S., 31
Maultsby, Maxie, 98
Moore, Bob, 51, 52, 102
Multimodal Life History Questionnaire, 41
'must', 86

negative emotions
    healthy and unhealthy, 13, 28–29
Neimark, P., 116
neurotic agreement, 128–129
Nolen-Hoeksema, S., 73, 108
non-verbal behaviour, 24–25

obsessive–compulsive personality, 40
obstacles to client change, 107–109

overlearning
    encouraging use of, 102–103

pacing, 9
panic disorder, 30–31
paraverbal behaviour, 24–25
philosophical change, 16
pragmatic disputes, 87–88
problem list, 44–45, 118
problem specificity, 46
Problems and Goals rating scales, 68

questions
    flexibility in, 49–50
    open-ended versus theory-derived, 50
    use of, 48–50

'rational'
    different meanings of, 13
rational alternatives
    encouragement of, 96–97
rational beliefs
    versus irrational beliefs, 27–28
    undermining of, 112
rational emotive behavioural treatment sequence, 44–45, 47, 57
referrals, 115–116
reflective process, 12, 110
reinforcement of change, 59
relapse prevention, 33–34
repetition
    therapist, 60
resignation
    versus acceptance, 32–33
responsibility
    client assumption of, 65–66
    teaching of emotional, 25–26
review sessions, 12, 21–22

Safran, J.D., 3
Schneiman, R.S., 115
self-acceptance, 119–120
self-disclosure (therapist), 5
self-downing beliefs, 27
    disputing of, 94–95
self-help
    daily assignments, 76–77
    forms, 67–74
    non-completion of assignments, 75–76
    in therapy, 35

self-help forms, 67–71, 74, 78
  training clients to use, 71–73
self-supervision, 130–131
self-therapy
  REBT, 35–36
shame, 55
socratic questioning, 49–50
  disputing, 88–89
structural life history questionnaire, 41
supervision, 129–130
  self-, 130–131

tangential talking, 42–43
tape-recording of sessions, 21–22
  supervision and, 130
target problem
  switching from the, 47–48
task assignment form, 71
tasks, 3
  change-producing, 66–67
  information for, 40–42
teaching styles, 7
technical issues, 39–62
techniques
  creation of new REBT, 121–122
temporary termination, 62
tennis
  rational and irrational, 119
termination of therapy
  flexibility in, 61–62
  temporary, 62
therapeutic alliance, 3–18
  use of concept of, 3–4
therapeutic arenas
  and REBT, 17–18
therapeutic style, 23

therapist
  challenge, 11
  defensiveness, 129
  directiveness, 8
  explanations to clients, 24
  humour, 5–6
  influence base of, 6–7
  insensitivity, 57–58
  interpersonal style of, 4–6
  irrational beliefs of, 127–128
  lack of skill of, 3, 8
  likeability, 7
  personal use of REBT, 131–132
  repetition, 60
  self-care of, 132–133
  self-development, 127–133
  self-disclosure, 5
therapy sessions
  fifty-minute hour, 116
  flexibility in, 116–117
  organisation/structure in, 39–40
  transcription of, 130–131
time-limited irrationalities, 55–57, 93
time-tripping imagery
  in disputing, 93

vivid interventions, 120–121

Walker, Jane, 68, 69
Weinrach, S.G., 132
Wessler, R.A., 51, 119, 130
Wessler, R.L., 51, 119, 130
working through of problems, 47–48

Yankura, J., 131
Young, Howard, 10, 91